Caring for the Older Person

Caring for the Older Person

Practical Care in Hospital, Care Home or at Home

ANN BRADSHAW RGN, DipN (Lond), PhD
Oxford Brookes University, School of Health and Social Care,
and Oxford Radcliffe Hospitals NHS Trust, Department of Clinical Geratology

CLAIR MERRIMAN RGN, BSc (Hons), MSc, Cert ed
Oxford Brookes University, School of Health and Social Care

John Wiley & Sons, Ltd

Copyright © 2007   John Wiley & Sons Ltd
The Atrium, Southern Gate, Chichester,
West Sussex PO19 8SQ, England
Telephone   (+44) 1243 779777

Email (for orders and customer service enquiries): cs-books@wiley.co.uk
Visit our Home Page on www.wiley.com

Other Wiley Editorial Offices

John Wiley & Sons Inc., 111 River Street, Hoboken, NJ 07030, USA

Jossey-Bass, 989 Market Street, San Francisco, CA 94103-1741, USA

Wiley-VCH Verlag GmbH, Boschstr. 12, D-69469 Weinheim, Germany

John Wiley & Sons Australia Ltd, 42 McDougall Street, Milton, Queensland 4064, Australia

John Wiley & Sons (Asia) Pte Ltd, 2 Clementi Loop #02-01, Jin Xing Distripark, Singapore 129809

John Wiley & Sons Canada Ltd, 6045 Freemont Blvd, Mississauga, ONT, L5R 4J3

Wiley also publishes its books in a variety of electronic formats. Some content that appears in print may
not be available in electronic books.

Anniversary Logo Design: Richard J. Pacifico

Library of Congress Cataloguing-in-Publication Data

Bradshaw, Ann.
    Caring for the older person : practical care in hospital, care home, or at home / by Ann Bradshaw,
Clair Merriman.
        p. ; cm.
    Includes bibliographical references and index.
    ISBN-13: 978-0-470-02563-5 (alk. paper)
    ISBN-10: 0-470-02563-8 (alk. paper)
    Older people–Medical care.   2. Older people–Hospital care.   3. Home care services.
    I. Merriman, Clair.   II. Title.
    [DNLM: 1. Geriatric Nursing–methods.   2. Aged.   WY152 B812c 2007]
    RA564.8.C374 2007
    649.8084′6–dc22

                                        2006028043

A catalogue record for this book is available from the British Library

ISBN-10: 0-470-02563-8
ISBN-13: 978-0-470-02563-5

Typeset by Techbooks, Delhi, India
Printed and bound in Great Britain by TJ International Ltd, Padstow, Cornwall

This book is printed on acid-free paper responsibly manufactured from sustainable forestry in which at
least two trees are planted for each one used for paper production.

Contents

Acknowledgements

We would like to thank Vicky MacArthur for her help and expertise in writing Chapter 3, 'Care for the older person requiring assistance with movement'. We would like to thank Allan MacArthur for taking the photographs and Anthony Knipe for preparing the symbols and diagrams that appear in the book. We would also like to thank Norgine for the use of the Movicol, Bristol Stool Form Scale.

A special thanks to Susan Lucksford for agreeing to appear in the photographs with Vicky MacArthur and Clair Merriman.

Introduction

REASON FOR THE BOOK

The aim of this book is to help you to develop the skills you need to care for older people, people over the age of 65. In British society older people are a growing proportion of the population. Since the 1930s the number of people over the age of 65 has doubled, and now make up one fifth of the population. Between 1995 and 2025 the number of people over 80 is set to increase by a half and the number of people over 90 will double. In hospital almost two thirds of beds are occupied by people over 65 (DoH 2001a).

This book starts with the requirements of the older person in need of care. It is written for anyone who is a practical carer of an older person, and who would like to learn the techniques and procedures necessary for care. You may be a health care professional or you may be a family member or friend, and the older person you are caring for may be in hospital, or at home or in a community nursing home.

The book has developed from the authors' own experiences as registered nurses and nurse teachers, and our own interests in caring for older people. Ann Bradshaw is concerned with the underlying ethos and values of care and, as part of this, how nurses achieve competence in care. Clair Merriman has a particular interest in developing a framework for teaching clinical skills to nursing students and registered nurses who need to maintain and update their competence. In addition, both authors have personal experience of caring for older family members. We have been helped in preparing this book by Vicky MacArthur, who is a qualified trainer in moving and handling procedures. In this book we aim to offer a systematic step-by-step approach to the fundamental care needs that an older person may have, and the procedural steps you as a carer might take to address these needs. Up-to-date evidence provides the rationale.

It is hoped this will be a useful resource not only for professional training purposes, if you are learning to be a nurse or care assistant, but also if you are caring for a friend or relative at home. As it is now recognised (DoH 2001a) that to be in one's own home for as long as possible leads to the best quality of life for the individual, it is hoped that this book will be of some assistance in furthering this aim and giving you confidence in caring for the older person. To simplify terms, the book will refer to the person who cares as 'the carer', whether you are a trained or untrained paid professional or a lay carer.

In twenty-first-century Britain, paid care is often delivered by people who are not nurses. This is likely to continue as professional boundaries in health care become less fixed (Wanless 2002). But such changes require appropriate training. The competent

registered nurse should supervise and monitor such training, and remains profession-
ally responsible and accountable for the care given (NMC 2004a).

It should be obvious that older people are not a homogeneous group. Each person
will have different health needs, concerns and personal circumstances, reflecting an
individual personal story. The requirement to ensure that the older person receives
care that is tailored to his or her personal needs, and that individuality is respected and
protected, is reflected in government policy. Policy documents such as *The National
Service Framework for Older People*, *Caring for Older People: a Nursing Priority*
and *The Essence of Care* (DoH 2001a, 2001b, 2001c) have sought to address this.
The need is summarised thus:

> In summary, older persons are the least satisfied with acute care of all age groups. The
> care they receive often fails to meet their most basic needs for food, fluid, rest, activity
> and elimination, let alone meeting their psychological needs. Current standards of care
> do not foster older people's sense of independence and self-direction and their dignity
> and self-respect is undermined. Nurses do not feel trained, supported or empowered to
> act as older person advocates and even within the profession, the nursing care of older
> people is seen as low status occupation. (DoH 2001b: p. 7, para 2.6)

This was written in 2001, but even five years later the need to improve care for
older people is still an important concern. *Living Well in Later Life* (Commission
for Healthcare Audit and Inspection 2006) found a lack of dignity and respect in the
way older people were treated while in hospital. This has been responded to by the
government with a document detailing the next steps in implementing the National
Service Framework for Older People *A New Ambition for Old Age* (DoH 2006). That
older people should be respected and cared for according to individual need is the
premise of this book.

KEEPING HEALTHY AND INDEPENDENT IN OLDER AGE: BACKGROUND AND UNDERLYING ASSUMPTIONS

The aim of all care is to help the older person maintain his or her health and independence as far as this is realistic and possible. This may mean regaining health
and independence after an illness. People differ in the way they age, and older age
cannot be defined neatly at a certain year of life. Nevertheless, while it is difficult to
define a person by their age, illness in later life has certain characteristics for all older
people. In later years people tend to suffer from more than one cause of ill health.
Illnesses tend to be more difficult to diagnose, older people may deteriorate rapidly
if untreated and have a higher incidence of complications. Disease in later life is
vulnerable to adverse environments. Practical care needs should be directed towards
active rehabilitation rather than just convalescence (Grimley Evans et al. 2000).

Ageing brings with it a progressive loss of adaptability for the older person. There
is a reduction in maximal performance as well as functional reserve. It requires more

effort for the older person just to maintain his or her activities of daily living (often called ADLs) than it does for the younger person. The gap between what the person is able to do and what he or she has to do, just to keep functioning in daily life, narrows. Hence the older person needs to work at maintaining this functional capacity. Ideally the older person should keep active in all daily activities of living such as shopping, cooking and washing in order to remain independent as far as this is possible. The practical need is to maintain a careful balance between promoting the older person's functional capacity and giving the person help when needed, even for a short time. If the older person does not use some capacity, for example as a result of illness, this may be recoverable initially but over time disuse will become permanent (Grimley Evans et al. 2000).

Because convalescence after illness takes longer than in younger people, early rehabilitation is vital, and needs to take into account the older person's home environment. Rehabilitation is unlike convalescence because it involves more than just spontaneous recovery. Rehabilitation changes the natural history of recovery so that it takes time, skilled people and adequate equipment. There needs to be a rapid response to illness with a full medical investigation by the doctor. A social and functional assessment involves the nurse, occupational therapist, physiotherapist and social worker. The older person may also need swallowing and nutritional assessments by speech and language therapist and dietitian, as well as assessment of sight, hearing and care of feet. Whether the older person experiences pain also needs to be considered, as this will affect movement and rehabilitation. Involvement of the multiprofessional team is vital (Grimley Evans et al. 2000). Hence, assessment should consider the medical prognosis and physical and mental function, including health habits, vision, hearing, motivation and cognitive status. Health care tools such as the Barthel Scale, Waterlow Score, Body Mass Index, Abbreviated Mental Test, Mini Mental State Examination, Geriatric Depression Scale and Malnutrition Universal Screening Tool may be used in assessment by members of the multiprofessional team.

But assessment also involves more than this. Assessment needs to provide information about how the older person is managing in daily life. Functional assessment develops a picture of what the person is capable of doing, how much help is needed, and what interventions can be made to maximise independence and safety (Sheehan 1997). Elements of functional assessment are varied but usually include questions about ADLs such as transferring from bed to chair, dressing, washing, toileting, eating and maintaining continence. Observation is also an important part of assessment, for example by watching the older person walk, get up from a chair, or perhaps get dressed. Instrumental activities of daily living (often called IADLs) include shopping for food, managing finances, driving and arranging transport, using the telephone, cleaning and laundry, housing issues.

In assessing the older person's care needs at home, the physical environment and involvement of family and friends also require consideration (Caird & Grimley Evans 1995). They may play a very important role in keeping the older person as active as possible. Activity, both physical and mental, not only raises the morale and spirits of the older person, but it improves rehabilitation at every level.

According to Grimley Evans et al. (2000) defined care objectives need to be set following assessment. These should reflect what the older person wants, and whether this is attainable, taking account both of the minimum requirements and of maximum achievements. Carers' views and available resources must be taken account of, and any necessary compromise needs to be negotiated. There should be a management plan involving carers about how care will be managed, taking account of what it will involve, when it should be done and by whom. It is also important to close the gap between the demands of the environment and the capabilities of the individual. This may be assisted by therapeutic interventions that improve function, such as lifestyle changes and medical treatments. It may also be helped by prosthetic interventions to reduce demands of the environment, by aids and adaptations and personal help from family, friends or services.

In order to hasten recovery from illness the older person needs to use reserve function and be motivated. Tasks should be simplified and muscles strengthened. Mechanisms of recovery will also include the learning of new manoeuvres. Underpinning rehabilitation are certain principles. The older person should be helped to maintain normality and avoid becoming dependent or take on a 'sick role'. Activities should be relevant to future needs and should be purposeful. In promoting rehabilitation frequent short episodes are more effective than fewer, longer ones. Praise for achievement is more effective than criticism for failure.

Finally, the rehabilitation of the older person needs to be reviewed regularly. The review should consider whether progress is expected. If it is not, it should be considered whether some factor, such as depression, demotivation, drug effects or new illness has intervened. A new plan may need to be established, and perhaps an audit should consider why the plan was wrong. Follow-ups need to check on progress in all aspects of rehabilitation and care.

PREVENTING FALLS IN THE OLDER PERSON

One of the common reasons why the older person loses his or her independence is as a result of a fall. When caring for the older person it is important that you have some knowledge of the assessment and prevention of falls. According to Help the Aged (2005) about a third of all people aged over 65 fall each year with higher rates among people over 75. Of this group, falls represent over half of hospital admissions for accidental injury, particularly hip fracture. Half of those people who have a hip fracture never regain their former level of function and one in five dies within three months. So it is important you are aware of strategies to prevent the older person for whom you are caring from falling.

When you assess the older person for whom you are caring, you should ask if he or she has fallen in the last year, and you should find out the frequency, context and characteristics of the fall. You should observe the older person's balance and gait, including appropriate footwear, as well as any weaknesses or impairments of movement, feeling, memory or vision. Consider too whether the older person is afraid of falling, has any continence problems or other functional problems, or whether he or she is taking many different medicines. You could also look for any hazards in the older person's environment (National Institute for Clinical Excellence 2004). In the home these might be loose rugs, slippery floors or trailing flexes. In hospital or care home this might also be equipment. Strength and balance training may help the older person avoid falling, so too may the removal of hazards, a review of medicines and treatments for heart irregularities. And as Help the Aged (2005) point out, most older people accept risk as a part of life. It is important that the carer is not overly prescriptive or patronising in any aspect of care.

PRACTICAL AIDS AND EQUIPMENT: FACILITATING INDEPENDENT LIVING

There are many practical aids to help the older person live at home and as independently as possible. The general practitioner or district nurse is the first port of call to explain what assistance is available to meet individual needs, and how it may be funded. The local social services and voluntary agencies such as Help the Aged and Age Concern will also have very helpful information about entitlements, assessments for these entitlements, and how they can best be provided and by whom.

On a practical level, it is important to know what aids are available – such as mobility aids, stair lifts, bath equipment, hand rails, door-answering devices, alarms, telephones with amplifiers and enlarged dials, devices that make handling cutlery or opening medicines easier, Internet adapting devices, and so on. These can now be purchased from high street stores and pharmacies as well as from specialist agencies. There are also services available such as continence delivery services, food delivery services, including businesses that deliver meals, and supermarkets that organise home delivery through the Internet. All these will help the older person maintain his or her own independent living.

Where more help is needed there are various statutory, private and voluntary agencies that may provide carers, offering different levels of care from nursing care to companionship. There may also be respite care available so that a family or friend carer can take a break.

THE FOCUS OF THE BOOK: ATTENDING TO THE PRACTICAL DETAILS OF CARE

While emphasising the importance of promoting health, independence and rehabilitation for the older person, the focus of this book is deliberately narrow, directed towards the older person who needs help. It is not the authors' intention to focus on specific disabilities or diseases; rather, this book concentrates on very specific practical tasks. These are fundamental to all other aspects of care. Indeed, systematic procedures do not preclude individualised care, but, rather, offer a sound basis for developing individualised care. Medical experts confirm that this attention to detail is the cornerstone of care for older people: 'Good quality medical and nursing care for older people requires scrupulous attention to detail since even the smallest error of judgement or lack of observation may have serious consequences for the older person' (Caird & Grimley Evans 1995, p. 4334).

CARING FOR THE WHOLE PERSON AND THE NEED FOR COMPASSION

It cannot be overstated that respect for the person, irrespective of age, is fundamental, so that needs should be attended to as immediately as is possible and, if necessary, explanations given for failures to do so. The essence of care should be centred on the older person as a person. This is the meaning of whole-person care, commonly now termed 'holistic' or 'person-centred' care – to see the person with all his or her history, relationships, hopes and fears.

Finally, it is important to note that this book cannot cover the most important aspect of care, that is, that the attitude of the carer towards the individual older person is crucial. It can be stated, for example, that the older person's arm should be lifted, but not stated how. Kindness, patience, gentleness, sensitivity, understanding and compassion are vital qualities for the carer, but this book can do no more than state the practical procedure.

However, the practicalities of care cannot be learned adequately from books, but need some form of apprenticeship training, by observing, watching and learning how it can be done. It is hoped that this book will be used in this way, and as a contribution to a careful way of care.

DISCLAIMER

The procedures detailed in this book are not definitive, as knowledge constantly changes. Medical and nursing knowledge is evolving, particularly with regard to treatment, procedures, equipment and drugs. While the authors and publisher have, as far as possible, ensured the information in the text is accurate and up-to-date, readers are strongly advised to confirm this information with the latest legislation and standards for practice. Because evidence is constantly changing there is a responsibility on the carer and his or her supervisor or trainer to ensure that the carer has the necessary knowledge of the relevant discipline as well as the skill needed to carry out the procedure. **It is important for the carer to get expert supervision, help and advice. The carer should not perform any procedures if not trained or competent to do so.**

As the Royal College of Nursing Institute (1998) states in the introduction to *Clinical Practice Guidelines*, in all clinical guidelines recommendations may not be appropriate for use in all circumstances. This is because a limitation of any guideline is that it simplifies clinical decision-making processes and recommendations. Decisions to adopt any particular recommendation or procedure must be made by the practitioner or carer in the light of available resources, local services, policies and protocols, the particular older person's circumstances and wishes, available personnel and equipment, clinical experience of the practitioner and knowledge of more recent research findings. The qualified health care practitioner is responsible and accountable for all care, even that which is delegated (NMC 2004a).

THE STRUCTURE OF THE BOOK

The book is divided into seven chapters. Chapter 1 describes the prerequisites of care, the essential requirements that underpin all care for the older person. Chapter 2 addresses personal cleansing requirements that the older person may have. Chapter 3 addresses the movement needs of the older person. Chapter 4 considers the older person who requires help with eating and drinking. Chapter 5 looks at how to help the older person who has toileting needs. Chapter 6 considers the older person whose condition necessitates observation and monitoring. The focus of Chapter 7 is the older person who is dying. Each chapter is further subdivided into a number of procedures. This is in order to cover a wide spectrum of fundamental needs. This should make it easy for you to select and tailor an individual plan of care for the older person for whom you are caring.

Health care professionals are responsible for ensuring that care is based on current evidence, best practice and, where applicable, validated research that is available (NMC 2004a). Hence, procedures detailed in each section will be referenced according to up-to-date evidence. The full reference list is given at the end of the book. References are not intended to be exclusive or definitive. The reference list is also useful for further reading.

Before you begin to plan your care by reading the book, you will need to read through the Preliminary Considerations and Symbols which focus on the fundamental aspects of care required for every procedure you will undertake.

1 Preliminary considerations and symbols

For ease and clarity, and to avoid repetition, symbols are used throughout this book. A symbol requires you to carry out an action. Each symbol is explained in this chapter. If you cannot remember how to carry out a certain activity, then please revisit the explanation of that particular symbol.

Whether you are a registered nurse, a student nurse, a health care assistant or a lay person, there are certain preliminary considerations that are important for the person you are caring for.

It cannot be overemphasised that before doing any procedure you should ensure that you have expert supervision, help and advice. You should not perform any procedure if not trained or competent to do so, or if you are in any doubt.

1. PREVENTING AND CONTROLLING INFECTION

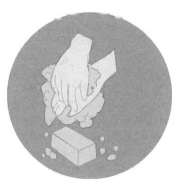

Symbol 1

STANDARD PRECAUTIONS

Everyone involved in providing care in the hospital or community needs to know about standard precautions, including hand decontamination and the use of protective clothing (gloves and aprons) (DoH 2001d, 2003). Standard precautions underpin safe practice, protecting both the carer and the older person from infection. Using standard precautions at all times will reduce the risks of cross-infection (RCN 2004).

HAND DECONTAMINATION

As a result of the ageing process the older person is particularly susceptible to developing infections. Hand decontamination is one of the most effective ways to prevent the spread of infection. Hands must be decontaminated immediately before and after each and every episode of person to person contact or any activity that could potentially result in your hands becoming contaminated (DoH 2001d, 2003). The following hand preparation increases the effectiveness of decontamination. Nails should be short, clean and polish-free, rings with ridges or stones should not be worn, and cuts and abrasions should be covered with a waterproof dressing (RCN 2004).

HAND WASHING

Hand washing is the single most important activity for reducing cross-infection (RCN 2004). Hands that are visibly soiled or grossly contaminated must be washed with liquid soap and water (DoH 2001d, 2003) (Table 1.1).

ALCOHOL HAND RUB AND ITS LIMITATIONS

Hands can be decontaminated with an alcohol-based hand rub in between activities if hands are visibly free from dirt (DoH 2003). If hands are not dirty to the naked eye, then alcohol is an excellent method for decontamination as long as it is used correctly (Storr & Clayton-Kent 2004) (Table 1.2). The Department of Health (2005a, 2005b) has pointed out that in the prevention and control of *Clostridium difficile* infection alcohol hand rub is insufficient as it does not kill all the spores. Therefore hand washing is essential if you are caring for the older person who is infected with *Clostridium difficile*.

PROTECTIVE CLOTHING

Protective clothing should be used to protect both you and the older person from the risks of cross-infection (DoH 2001d, 2003; RCN 2004). You will need to make a judgement as to what protective clothing is required based on a risk assessment of transmission of micro-organisms to the older person, and the risk of contamination to your clothing and skin by your older person's blood, body fluids, secretions or excretions (DoH 2001d, 2003). Protective clothing includes aprons and gloves.

NON-STERILE GLOVES

If gloves are to protect the carer then non-sterile gloves are normally the most appropriate (Workman & Bennett 2002). Sterile gloves should be worn for invasive procedures and contact with sterile sites. Non-sterile gloves should be used when there is non-intact skin or mucous membranes, and all activities that have been assessed as carrying a risk of exposure to blood, body fluids, secretions or excretions, or to sharp or contaminated instruments (Workman & Bennett 2002; Baillie 2005). They should also be used if the older person has an infection such as methicillin resistant *Staphylococcus aureus* (MRSA) or *Clostridium difficile*. It

Table 1.1 Preventing and controlling infection: hand washing

Procedure	Rationale
Stand in front of sink, ensuring hands and uniform/clothing do not touch the sink.	Inside of the sink is contaminated; touching the sink will contaminate hands and clothing.
Turn on the water and regulate so it does not splash and so temperature is warm.	If clothing is splashed it will provide an ideal place for micro-organisms to travel and grow. Warm water will remove less of the protective oils on the hands than hot water.
Wet hands and wrists thoroughly under running water and apply sufficient liquid soap to create a good lather.	Wetting skin prior to applying soap ensures that soap is diluted, and thus is less harsh to the skin.
Rub palm to palm, right palm over left dorsum, left palm over right dorsum, palm to palm, fingers interlaced, fingers to opposing palms, rotational rubbing of right thumb clasped over left palm and vice versa, rotational rubbing backwards and forwards with fingers of right hand in palm of left and vica versa. Rub at least five times at each step to ensure effective decontamination.	The mechanical action of rubbing helps to remove bacteria; this should be carried out for a minimum of 10–15 seconds. If the correct technique is not used many areas of the hands can be missed.
With fingers pointing upwards rinse hands until all traces of soap are removed, allowing the water to run down the hands.	Rinsing washes away dirt and micro-organisms.
Turn off taps with your foot or elbow. If the taps are not lever-operated or foot-operated use a paper towel to turn off the taps once your hands are dry.	To prevent re-contamination.
Dry your hands from fingers to wrist, using paper towels or a clean linen towel (community).	Using a wet paper towel will allow transfer of pathogens from the taps by capillary action. If hands are not dry the warm moisture is an ideal place for bacteria to grow. Paper towels are best practice for drying hands as they can further remove bacteria and lose dead skin cells. Linen towels can spread infection if not laundered in between each usage.
Discard the used paper towels or linen towel according to local policy, using a foot-operated waste bin.	Touching the bin lid with hands will cause re-contamination.
Handcream should be applied regularly from either a personal dispenser or hand pump device.	To protect the skin from drying due to regular decontamination and reduce bacterial growth and contamination between individuals.

Table 1.2   Preventing and controlling infection: hand decontamination using alcohol gel

Procedure	Rationale
Apply at least 5 ml of alcohol hand rub into palm of hands.	The hand rub needs to come into contact with all surfaces of the hands to ensure decontamination.
Rub palm to palm, right palm over left dorsum, left palm over right dorsum, palm to palm, fingers interlaced, fingers to opposing palms, rotational rubbing of right thumb clasped over left palm and vice versa, rotational rubbing backwards and forwards with fingers of right hand in palm of left and vice versa.	To ensure that all areas of the hand are decontaminated.
Continue to rub until solution has evaporated and hands are dry.	If hands are not dry the warm moisture is an ideal place for bacteria to grow.
Handcream should be applied regularly from either a personal dispenser or hand pump device.	To protect the skin from drying due to regular decontamination and reduce bacterial growth and contamination between individuals.

is recommended that seamless, single-use latex or vinyl gloves are used. Research shows that latex gloves offer more protection than vinyl or polythene gloves (Johnson 1997; O'Toole 1997; Ross 1999). However, if either the older person or carer is sensitive to latex this should be documented and alternatives should be provided and worn (DoH 2003). Non-sterile gloves fit either hand and are available in three sizes – small, medium or large. It is important that you use the correct size for you, otherwise dexterity will be compromised (Nicol et al. 2005).

Gloves are a single-use item, and therefore should be put on immediately before an episode of person-to-person contact or treatment and removed as soon as the activity is completed (DoH 2003; RCN 2004; Nicol et al. 2005). Gloves should be changed between different tasks of care for the same person, and when caring for different older persons (DoH 2003). Used gloves must be disposed of into the clinical waste (DoH 2003; Nicol et al. 2005). Gloves do not provide a substitute for hand washing, but are used to protect carers and older persons from cross-infection. They provide a warm, moist environment that encourages bacteria to grow and may be penetrated by external bacteria. It is essential that hands are decontaminated prior to putting gloves on and following removal of them (Workman & Bennett 2002; DoH 2003).

APRONS

Plastic aprons provide a barrier between the older person and carer's clothing and thus help to reduce cross-infection. Disposable plastic aprons should be worn whenever there is a risk of contaminating clothing or carer's skin with blood, body fluids, secretions or excretions and when an older person has a known infection such as MRSA (DoH 2001d, 2003; RCN 2004). Plastic aprons should be worn as single-use items, for one procedure or episode of older person care and then discarded or changed as deemed necessary (DoH 2003). Hands should be decontaminated prior to putting an apron on and following removal of apron. If gloves are also required, these should be put on after the apron and removed before the apron is removed (Nicol et al. 2005). When removing the apron, pull at the top and sides to break the neckband and waist ties and fold it in on itself to prevent the spread of micro-organisms on to your uniform or clothing (Workman & Bennett 2002; Nicol et al. 2005). Once the apron is removed it needs to be disposed of as clinical waste (Workman & Bennett 2002; DoH 2003; Nicol et al. 2005).

WASTE DISPOSAL

Waste is divided into two categories: non-clinical (domestic) and clinical waste. A colour-coding system for waste bags has been adopted nationally (Health and Safety Executive, Health Services Advisory Committee 1992). Uncontaminated waste that is generated either in hospitals or in homes can be disposed of in the same way as normal household waste. This includes paper towels, newspapers, dead flowers, food packaging. Normally this will be a black bag, but you will need to refer to local policies.

Clinical waste is anything that unless rendered safe may prove hazardous to any person coming into contact with it. Clinical waste means any waste which consists wholly or partly of:

• human tissue
• blood or other body fluids, for example wound drains, catheter bags
• excretions
• drugs or other pharmaceutical products
• swabs or dressings
• used aprons and gloves.

All clinical waste needs to be placed into the correct bag, usually a yellow bag, but once again you will need to refer to your local policies. If you are caring for someone in the community you will need to seek guidance from your District Nurse or GP, as in England and Wales certain categories of clinical waste such as urine containers or incontinence pads can be landfilled if a site is licensed for this use (Phillips 1999). Clinical waste bags should be separated from other waste. If leakage of bodily fluids is likely to occur, a second bag or container should be used to prevent exposure to and possible contamination of those who handle the waste products. Clinical waste bags need to be tied and sealed once they are two thirds full, as overfilling can cause waste to leak out. They also need to be labelled with the point of origin in order to identify the source if problems arise during disposal (Health and Safety Executive, Health Services Advisory Committee 1992).

SAFE DISPOSAL OF SHARPS

Sharps include needles, staples, stitch cutters, glass ampoules and any sharp instrument. To reduce the risk of injury and exposure to blood-borne viruses it is vital that sharps are used safely and are disposed of carefully. The main hazards of a sharps injury are hepatitis B, hepatitis C and HIV. You will need to follow your local policies and guidelines; both hospitals and community health centres will have clear polices on the disposal of sharps used in hospital and the older person's home. If you need to use sharps while caring for the older person you should take responsibility for any sharps used and dispose of them in a designated container at the point of use. The container should conform to UN standard 3291 and British Standard 7320 (RCN 2004). Sharp containers, normally yellow with a red lid, are rigid, puncture-resistant and leak-proof. They have a special opening which is designed to allow sharps to be dropped easily into the container. To prevent the risk of injury, sharps bins should not be overfilled. Thus it is recommended that they be sealed once they are three quarters full. You will need to seal the containers according to the manufacturer's instructions, label with date and source, and then leave for collection according to local policy guidelines.

The following are pointers that can help reduce the risk of a sharps injury:

- Do not pass sharps from hand to hand.
- Keep handling to a minimum.
- Do not break or bend needles before use or disposal.
- Do not dismantle syringes or needles by hand, and dispose of them as a single unit.
- Never re-sheath needles.
- Use sharps trays with integral sharps bins.
- Dispose of sharps at the point of use.

2.   CLEAR COMMUNICATION AND CONSENT TO CARE

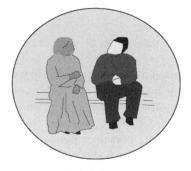

Symbol 2

Communication is an exchange, between a minimum of two people, of facts, needs, opinions, thoughts, feelings or other information by both verbal and non-verbal means (DoH. 2001b). One of the key elements of communication is that individuals should receive comprehensive information about all aspects of their care so that informed consent can be obtained.

Prior to caring for or treating the older person you need to make sure you have the person's consent (this involves anything you do, from helping the older person get dressed to giving him or her medication). Respecting the person's rights is not only a fundamental part of good practice but also a legal requirement (DoH 2001e, 2001f). Any person has the right to accept or refuse treatment or care if they have the capacity to do so. It should never be assumed that the older person is not able to make his or her own decisions simply because of age and frailty. The Department of Health (2001d, 2001f) guidelines are clear on consent. No one else is able to give consent on behalf of another adult. While it is important to communicate with close family members or friends – if that is what the older person would like – the need to respect autonomy in decision-making of the older person is essential.

For consent to be valid the older person must be competent to take that decision, must be acting voluntarily, and should have enough information to enable him or her to make the decision. The presumption is that the older person is mentally competent unless this is rebutted by evidence to the contrary. According to Dimond (2005, p. 144) a person lacks capacity to give a valid consent

> if some impairment or disturbance of mental functioning renders the person unable to make a decision whether to consent to or refuse treatment. That inability to make a decision will occur when:
>
> a) The patient is unable to comprehend and retain the information which is material to the decision, especially as to the likely consequences of having or not having the treatment in question.
> b) The patient is unable to use the information and weigh it in the balance as part of the process of arriving at the decision.

Seeking consent is a fundamental part of a therapeutic relationship and should be seen as a process, not as a one-off event. Legally, consent does not have to be written, and for aspects of care such as washing and dressing verbal consent is normally obtained. Prior to giving consent older persons require enough information in order for them to make an informed decision. In particular the older person will need to be aware of the benefits and the risks of the proposed treatment, what the treatment will involve, what the implications of not having the treatment are and what alternatives may be available. It is essential that this information is provided in a format that the older person can understand.

If the older person is not competent to make a decision, for example because he or she has dementia, the 'reasonable person' rule is applied. This enables a professional to act in the 'best interests' of the older person, thus allowing them to carry out interventions that are in the older person's best interest. Carers have a moral obligation to do no harm (non-maleficence) and to promote good (beneficence) (Beauchamp & Childress 2001). This implies that they need to balance the risks with the benefits associated with all forms of care. This can be a very difficult decision to make, and sometimes needs to be made rapidly. It may be difficult to keep in balance the need to promote the older person's independence, while at the same time protecting him or her from harm. Involve family and colleagues in complex decisions.

Holistic care

X

Communicating with the older person is fundamental to every aspect of care, from assessing needs, planning how to address those needs, implementing a plan of care and evaluating whether needs are being addressed and met. It is also crucial for the building up of a trusting relationship between the person caring, and the person being cared for. At every stage procedures of care should be fully explained to and discussed with the older person.

As people grow older hearing and sight may become less acute and so hinder communication. The older person may have some sensory impairment such as difficulty seeing or hearing (Coni & Webster 1998). Spectacles should be kept near the person, in a clean condition and their effectiveness regularly checked. Glare should be avoided and lighting should be appropriate. Large-print leaflets and books, or taped books and newspapers may also be useful. Sensitive touch may help communication with the visually impaired person. If the older person has a hearing aid, it should be correctly inserted, maintained and operated. Ear-wax can blur hearing, but should only be removed by a trained person. Background noise should be eliminated as far as possible. When speaking to the older person it is important for the older person to see the speaker's face and lips. The speaker should not shout but speak slowly and clearly without exaggerating words. The older person should be asked if they can hear, and if necessary words can be written down.

3. MAINTAINING THE PERSON'S PRIVACY, DIGNITY AND COMFORT

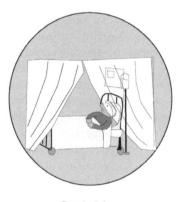

Symbol 3

Paying attention to the older person's dignity, privacy and comfort is fundamental to care and preserving the older person's personal identity. The context of care should actively respect the older person, his or her values, beliefs, personal relationships and personal preferences (DoH 2001b). If it is your first meeting with the older person, introduce yourself and ask how the older person would like to be addressed. To maintain the older person's privacy is to ensure that he or she is free from intrusion as far as possible, that personal boundaries and space are protected, and that he or she feels that they matter at all times.

Think in advance what you will need for each procedure, so that before any procedure you ensure that all equipment is collected and ready. This will avoid leaving the older person, in the middle of a procedure, to collect equipment. Privacy, dignity and modesty are protected by using screens, curtains and closing doors when appropriate, and by keeping the older person's body covered with a sheet, blanket or clothing while carrying out procedures. Whenever possible, ensure the older person's elimination and hygiene needs are met in an appropriate place, for example the bathroom or toilet. Make sure you maintain the older person's comfort by giving spectacles, hearing aids, access to drink, call bell, tissues, newspaper, book, television control and so on, prior to leaving the older person. Choice in clothing is crucial. In hospital or care home, especially, it is important that the older person has his or her own clothes.

As part of maintaining the older person's privacy, protecting confidentiality is very important. This should be maintained by only sharing information when necessary and protecting information from improper disclosure. This is a requirement for health care professionals (NMC 2004a), but it is also important for the lay carer. Before any information about the older person is shared with another health care professional, or family member, the older person's permission should always be sought. If the older person is incapable of giving such permission, ask for professional advice from other health care professionals in the best interests of the older person.

4. KEEPING RECORDS AND DOCUMENTING CARE

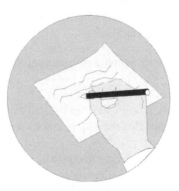

Symbol 4

Every older person should have an individualised care plan. A nursing care plan is a written, structured plan of action for care. It involves four steps: assessment, planning, implementation and evaluation. A care plan should provide an appropriate method of monitoring and assessing the older person's progress effectively, as well as detailing nursing treatment and care provided. Wherever practicable it should be written with the involvement of the older person.

Prior to providing any care you should read the care plan, and any other relevant records available to you, to get as full a picture as possible of the older person, his or her specific needs, issues that have affected care previously, and any proposed future plans of care, including what may be considered to be effective and ineffective. Before you start you will need to assess how care can best be carried out so that independence is promoted. Any plan of care should also aim at meeting the requirements of the *National Service Framework for Older People* (DoH 2001a).

Record keeping is a professional requirement of all health care professionals in the UK, who must draw up and maintain records of all care. These records are legal documents and it is therefore essential that they are maintained accurately and neatly and include recordings of vital signs, pressure-sore prevention scores, fluid balance charts, food charts and so on. Good record keeping promotes high standards and continuity of care, better communication between health care professionals, an accurate account of care planning and delivery, and the ability to detect at an early stage problems such as changes in the older person's condition (NMC 2004b).

If a written care plan is crucial for the professional carer it is also extremely useful for the lay carer for the same reasons. It will help provide a framework and structure for the care to be given, provide a record and reminder of the care that has been given, what has been achieved and any problems or needs still to be addressed. It will highlight at an early stage changes in the older person's condition. It can also be used as a tool of communication for the older person being cared for, other carers and health care professionals.

The following points from the Nursing and Midwifery Council's *Guidelines for Records and Record Keeping* (NMC 2004b) offer some important tips to ensure that your documentation is of a high standard:

- The record contains a clear account of nursing treatment and nursing care provided.
- The record is factual, consistent and accurate.
- The record has been clearly written and can be easily read by others.
- The record is written in terms that the older person can easily understand.
- The record is written in ink.
- The record does not include abbreviations, jargon, meaningless phrases, irrelevant speculation or offensive subjective statements.
- All alterations or additions are dated, timed and signed.
- All entries are dated, timed and signed.
- All entries should be written contemporaneously, or as soon as possible after care has been given.

5.   MOVING AND HANDLING

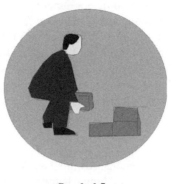

Symbol 5

The older person who is in need of care may well also require from the carer help to move. All carers involved in manual handling should have a practical understanding of the legislation relevant to this area (Mandelstam 2002). There are five pieces of legislation that govern Moving and Handling at work. These set out the legal responsibilities for the health care professional, and employers of health care professionals, in order that harm is not caused to either the carer or the person for whom he or she cares. It is also vitally important for the lay carer, for the very same reasons. Hence, you need to know about the legislation, and ways to protect both yourself and the older person for whom you are caring.

This legislation is as follows:

- The Health and Safety at Work Act (1974) (HASAW)
  This Act sets out employer and employee responsibilities in the workplace. Under this Act employers are responsible for the health, safety and welfare of their employees. They must provide instruction, supervision and training for them. Employees are responsible for their own health, safety and welfare and should cooperate with the employer to enable him or her to comply with his or her health and safety duties. This includes attending training offered, and working in the way you have been shown in this training.
- The Manual Handling Operations Regulations (1992) (MHOR)
  This directive came into force in January 1993. Hazardous manual handling operations must be avoided so far as is reasonably practicable. Where these operations cannot be avoided, a suitable and sufficient assessment must be made before the operation is carried out. The risk of injury from these operations must be reduced so far as is reasonably practicable.
- The Lifting Operations and Lifting Equipment Regulations (1998) (LOLER)
  This places requirements on organisations to ensure the safety and suitability of manual handling equipment. In particular, organisations must ensure that:

Lifting equipment is appropriate for the setting.

Lifting equipment is periodically checked and maintained.

Staff are trained in the use of lifting equipment.

Unsafe or broken lifting equipment is removed from use immediately.

- Provision and Use of Work Equipment Regulations (1998) (PUWER)
  These regulations cover all equipment used at work including moving and handling and lifting equipment. They impose a range of duties concerning matters such as: employers providing suitable work equipment; employers providing information, instruction and training for people who use work equipment; that equipment should be maintained in good repair and regularly inspected with records of inspections kept.
- Human Rights Act (1998)
  The European Convention on Human Rights has been incorporated into UK law since October 2000 by means of the Human Rights Act. There are a number of wide-ranging rights, three of which have potential application to Moving and Handling:

  Article 3: 'No one shall be subjected to ... inhuman or degrading treatment ... '
  Article 5: 'Everyone has the right to liberty and security of person.'
  Article 8: 'Everyone has the right to respect for his private and family life, his home and correspondence.'

  The greatest concern in terms of Moving and Handling in relation to this Act is the perceived conflict between the right of the person needing care to refuse to be handled in a certain way (for example, with a hoist), and the right of the carer to refuse to endanger themselves (by manually lifting as an alternative to hoisting). This does not mean that you are within your rights to refuse to manually handle people. Rather, you should aim for a balanced approach to protect both the carer and the person being cared for through risk assessment.
- Health care professionals also have a duty of care under the NHS Act 1977, NHS and Community Care Act 1990 and Care Standards Act 2000. These documents require health care professionals to assess need and meet identified needs as far as is practical.

RISK ASSESSMENT

A risk is a likelihood that harm will be realised. A risk assessment considers the probability of an incident occurring, the severity of the injury or damage that may occur and the steps needed to control the risk (HSC 1998). Undertaking risk assessments and acting on the recommendations is a legal obligation (Tracy 1999). The steps involved are: look at the hazards, that is, something with a potential to cause harm; decide who might be harmed and how; evaluate the risks and decide whether existing precautions are adequate; record your findings; finally, review your assessment and revise if necessary (HSC 1998).

Prior to undertaking any moving and handling operation you need to ask: Can I avoid moving or handling in this instance? Could the older person, with instruction or equipment, do it themselves? If not, then the risks involved must be assessed.

Table 1.3 Moving and handling: four factors of risk

1 THE LOAD	2 THE TASK
(the older person) Is he or she:	Does the task involve anything we know to be risky? Consider:
• heavy? • bulky? • difficult to grasp? • potentially dangerous?	• distance of load from trunk • twisting or stooping or a combination • excessive lifting, lowering or carrying distances • excessive pushing or pulling • likelihood of sudden movement • frequent or prolonged physical effort • rest or recovery periods • handling while seated • team handling

3 INDIVIDUAL CAPACITY	4 THE WORKING ENVIRONMENT
Of the person performing the manoeuvre, e.g. tired, unsure of how to use the equipment, stressed, pregnant, previous back injury? Does the task:	Are there:
• require strength, height, etc? • require special knowledge or training? • put at risk employees who are pregnant or have ill health?	• space constraints? • uneven, slippery floors? • varied levels of floors or surfaces? • extremes of temperature, humidity or air movement? • poor lighting?

(Adapted from Johnson 2005)

When assistance is needed, individual assessment of the older person is required. This, along with a strategy for moving and handling the person, must be recorded in the care plan and communicated to all staff. These should be updated regularly, or as required.

Every carer should also conduct an on-the-spot assessment prior to handling the older person, to judge their capabilities and any changes in his or her condition.

In assessing risk there are four factors to be considered. The acronym TILE helps us to remember these: task, individual capability, load and environment (RCN 2003). These are highlighted in Table 1.3. An answer of yes to any of these questions indicates a potential problem area.

Having considered the risks in the above areas, ways of reducing them must be identified. For example, breaking the task down into smaller components; making the load easier to grasp, for example with a handling belt; moving furniture to create more space. It is crucially important to be trained how to use any moving and handling equipment.

Ways that will help you break down the task into smaller components are listed in Table 1.4.

Table 1.4   Moving and handling: breaking the task down

LOAD	
Make it lighter	By gaining the older person's cooperation and maximum assistance, using handling aids and/or sharing the load with colleagues.
Make it easier to manage	Think through task and consider attachments such as intravenous lines and cardiac monitors.
Make it easier to grasp	Use handling belts.
Make it more stable	Consider possibility of unexpected movements by the older person and make advance provision, e.g. extra help.
Make it less damaging to hold	As above.
INDIVIDUAL CAPACITY	
Awareness of personal capacity	The right attitude
Provision of knowledge and training	The right knowledge
Staff selection appropriate for the task	The right skill
TASK	
Improving task layout	Reduce distances to be moved or break task down into several shorter moves.
Using the body more efficiently	Most transfers can be achieved with less exertion using a sliding aid.
Improving work routine	Rest breaks or less tiring spells of work introduced around the task.
Provision of training in handling while seated	
Provision of training in team handling	A team leader should be identified and clear commands should be agreed upon with the team and the older person. The command 'one, two three' should *not* be used. Instead 'ready, steady, go' is used. 'Go' can be changed to any appropriate action word such as 'slide', 'stand' or 'roll'.
Provision of personal protective equipment	Enabling you to get closer to the load.
Maintenance and accessibility of equipment	Does the hoist fit in the bathroom, etc.?
WORKING ENVIRONMENT	
Remove space constraints	All unnecessary furniture should be moved out of the way.
Consider nature and condition of floor	
Reduce work at different levels	Avoid stooping at all times.
Control thermal environment	
Maximise lighting conditions	Improve orientation of the older person to task.

ASSESSMENT OF THE OLDER PERSON

When manual handling is unavoidable, individual person assessment is required. This provides you with more information about your 'load' (the older person) when undertaking your risk assessment. When performing assessment of the older person, several factors need to be considered: the older person's ability to assist; any confusion or aggression; any limb or muscle weakness; any history of falls; skin condition; level of consciousness; any visual/hearing impairments; any attachments such as drips and drains; any pain.

SELECTING THE TECHNIQUE

Having considered the factors above, the carer must decide on one of four ways of carrying out the task. First, let the older person move himself or herself; second, use a sliding system; third, use a mechanical device or, fourth, do not do the task and review the analysis. Before using any sliding systems or mechanical devices you will need to make sure that you have been trained to use them and are competent to do so. The selected techniques should be communicated to the older person and any other carers, so that instructions are understood. The care plan should include information on the handling aids and techniques to be used and the number of carers required.

The initial assessment will need reviewing and updating as conditions change. Assessment is an on-going process. Having consulted the assessment, every carer still needs to do an on-the-spot assessment to determine if the plan is still appropriate and whether the carer and the older person are capable of executing the manoeuvre. Hence, avoid the need to manually handle someone if they could do it themselves with aids or encouragement. Assess the risk to you and the older person in what you are going to do. Reduce the risk to a reasonable level through the use of help and resources. Review the success of your intervention and re-assess if necessary.

PRINCIPLES FOR MANUAL HANDLING

There are three basic principles that you should remember to ensure that the techniques you use are safe both for you and for the older person (Centaur 1999).

1. Keep your spine in line. You may have been told at some time in life to 'keep your back straight'. In fact the spine is not straight but forms a natural S-shaped curve, with curves at the neck (cervical spine) and lower back (lumbar spine). When the spine is in this position it is 'at rest' and is able to recover from the stresses and strains put upon it by everyday movement. You should try to maintain this posture as often as possible through good standing and seated posture, allowing your back to recover between manual handling procedures. Raising your chin prior to any manoeuvre helps to align your spine.
2. Make a stable base. You make a stable base with your feet. The larger the base, the more stable you are. The largest base you can make is by tracing a reverse L-shape with your feet; stand with your feet together, move the right foot sideways

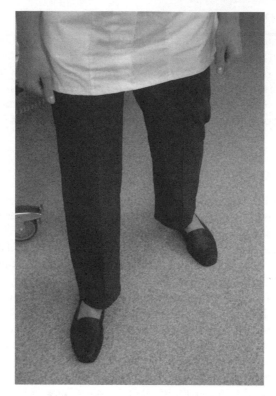

Figure 1.1

to hip distance apart, then move it forward. You can then keep your line of gravity (imagine a line running through the top of your head to the ground) within this base (Figure 1.1).
3. Short levers. Our levers are our arms. You should avoid extending your arms during manual handling procedures. In order to do this you should move close to the object to be handled, or, rather than bending at the waist to pick up an object, you should bend your knees.

DON'TS: UNSAFE TECHNIQUES

There are a number of techniques that are considered unsafe, both for the person being moved and the carer (Ruszala 2005). These are:

1. The drag lift. This is any technique that uses the person's arms as a 'handle'. The carers put their arms under the person's axilla (armpit) and pull them upwards. It might include pulling a person up in bed or the chair, or helping them to stand from a sitting position. Damage can be done to the older person's shoulder joint

and skin where it is being dragged against sheets and the carer is taking too much weight.

2. The orthodox or cradle lift. In this technique two carers join hands underneath the person's legs and back, facing each other across the bed. They then lift and swing the person up the bed to move them. The carers are in a poor position (arms extended and bending over) and are taking too much weight.

3. The Australian lift. This is a complicated lift that involves two carers. Two carers face the head of the bed and each places their nearest arm under the patient's legs and they join hands. The other hand is placed on the bed, or grasps the bed head. They kneel on the bed with the leg that is nearest the person, with the other foot on the floor. They place their nearest shoulder under the person's axilla and, by extending their legs, lift the person off the surface and move forward, up the bed. In this technique the carers are taking too much weight, and are kneeling on the bed, which can spread infection between beds. They are risking damage to the person's axilla as before.

4. The bear-hug/pivot. In this technique the carer allows the seated person to link arms either behind the carer's back, or, more dangerously, around their neck. The carer then links hands behind the person's back and pulls them up to a standing position. On reaching a standing position, the person and carer are in an unstable position and could fall. The carer is taking too much weight.

5. Through-arm lift. In this technique the carer, positioned behind the person, passes their arms underneath the axilla on each side and grasps the forearm of the person to be moved. They then lift the patient back into the chair or bed. This can be done with two carers, one on each side, or 'top and tail' with the second carer lifting the person's legs. They are risking damage to the person's axilla as before.

You should attend any moving and handling training that teaches the correct techniques that are safer for you and those you are caring for.

HOW TO USE THE SYMBOLS

Each procedure will start with the five symbols (see above). This is a reminder that you should observe them throughout the procedure, because they are fundamental prerequisites to care. You will need to use your own judgement and discretion about the emphasis you place on the particular symbol as you carry out the procedure. The information above will help you in making this decision. For example, preventing and controlling infection by handwashing will be relevant at various stages throughout any procedure. So you may need to wash your hands and change your gloves several times as you care for the older person.

It is important that you do not perform any procedure if you do not have the knowledge and skill to do so.

2 Care for the older person requiring assistance with personal cleansing

This chapter concerns personal and oral hygiene: cleansing the body to ensure that skin, hair, eyes, nails and mouth are maintained in an optimum condition, and that the physical environment is, and feels, clean and comfortable. The maintenance of cleanliness has been reinforced regularly by a number of nursing writers. Henderson and Nite (1978) suggest that personal hygiene is essential for maintenance of the older person's physical and mental state, while Roper, Logan and Tierney (1985) believe that hygiene habits are built into a routine which gives a pattern to the day, and provides the older person with security and stability. They follow in the tradition of Florence Nightingale (1860) who believed that cleanliness and hygiene, whether in sickness or in health, were fundamental to the well-being of the person.

These writers are supported more recently by the *National Service Framework for Older People* (DoH 2001a) and *The Essence of Care* benchmark for personal and oral hygiene (DOH 2001c). Both policy documents clearly state that all older people who need care should be assessed to identify the advice and/or care required to maintain and promote individual personal hygiene needs, including bathing. Intimate interventions should be met sensitively and respectfully and carried out in privacy so as to maintain the older person's dignity. In hospital, the older person should be enabled to wear his or her own clothes, if he or she so chooses, and have personal possessions around, if space allows. This supports the older person's integrity, and helps him or her feel more secure and so make the most of independence and mobility.

As the carer your first step is to assess the older person's individual personal and oral hygiene needs and his or her own capabilities in maintaining them. Assessment involves asking and discussing with the older person and their family what these needs are, observing the older person, and also examining nursing and medical records to ascertain any specific precautions about the older person's condition and care (Ochs & Castaldi 2001). In order to do this you should consider the older person's physical ability, the effect of any underlying diseases, and any particular risks such as infection. You will need to assess what the older person is able to do unaided and also what help they usually have and need.

The older person's expectations about cleanliness are based on family influences, peer groups, cultural differences, economic factors and social isolation. It is therefore important to take account of any personal preferences, or religious and cultural needs with regard to personal hygiene. If in hospital, the older person might like a family member to assist with washing and dressing; it is possible, however, that the older person or the family might feel uncomfortable with this kind of intimate involvement. Here again, as a carer you will need sensitivity to perceive and interpret what involvement in care the family would like.

Assessment will focus on the older person's ability to wash, dress, bathe, comb hair, clean teeth and dentures, clean spectacles and adjust and clean hearing aids. Communication and discussion with the older person needs to take account of his or her eyesight and hearing. You should negotiate and plan the older person's personal hygiene needs according to this assessment. This ensures that the older person receives care that is person-centred, that is, that takes into account the breadth and depth of the older person's life and relationships.

CARE OF SKIN AND HAIR

The skin is the largest organ of the body and makes up about 15 per cent of the total body weight (Penzer & Finch 2001; Hampton 2004). The natural ageing process affects the functions of the skin, and in particular makes the skin less able to withstand normal wear and tear. Therefore care of the skin of the older person should be an important aspect of overall care (Hampton 2004). As the skin ages it tends to become dry, thin and inelastic. Hair tends to thin and become more brittle. Moisturising creams are better for the skin than soap as soap has been found to raise the potential of skin tears in the older person (Birch & Coggins 2003). Soap substitutes such as aqueous cream can be used as an alternative, and have been found to be more effective and less time-consuming than using soap, water and moisturiser (Lewis-Byers & Thayner 2002). Although non-perfumed, bland products are best, if the older person likes a particular product this can be used unless adverse effects have been noted, such as allergies or sensitivities (Penzer & Finch 2001). Particular care should be taken to wash and dry the axillae, between the toes, the genital regions, and under the female's breasts, as all these areas are prone to becoming sore. Careful drying is important to prevent infection. The body takes longer to adjust to temperature so it is important to preserve the older person's warmth while he or she is washing, as well as to protect his or her dignity and privacy. If the older person wears cosmetics, you should ensure they are within reach, or help in applying them if required.

PREVENTION OF PRESSURE ULCERS

There are many factors in the development of pressure ulcers including illness, age, nutrition and hydration, position, shear and friction (RCN 2001). Skin should be inspected regularly for signs of pressure such as redness, discoloration and damage. You should check regularly over bony prominences: the ear, occiput, shoulder blades, spine, elbow, inside knee, heel and ankle, sacrum, iliac crest, hip. Pressure relieving devices, such as air mattresses and cushions, may assist in prevention. Further advice can be obtained from specialist nurses.

CARE OF NAILS

Care of nails is essential to maintaining a good quality of life for the older person and promoting independence (Papoola, Jenkins & Griffin 2005). In the older person nails become rigid, and thick. If not cared for they may grow inwards. You should carefully check toe and fingernails if the older person is unable to do this unaided. The older person who has visual difficulties, arthritis or stroke may not be able to maintain his or her nails, particularly toenails (Coni & Webster 1998). If the nails are dirty, cotton buds may be used to clean them. Unless the older person specifies otherwise, you should try and keep nails short by clipping them, being careful not to cut the skin. Toenails should be cut straight across rather than round. If the older person has diabetes, special care of the feet and toenails is required to prevent injury which may lead to foot ulceration. The older person with diabetes may experience reduced sensation and numbness in the feet. In this case, you should seek specialist advice from a podiatrist. If the older person likes to wear nail varnish you should ensure that this is within reach and help to apply or remove it, if required.

CARE OF EYES

One per cent of people over the age of 65 are registered partially sighted, and many more are visually disabled, although unregistered. Changes in sight may be caused by age, heredity, underlying disease such as hypertension and diabetes, as well as drugs such as steroids. In order to care for, and hence communicate with, the older person who is visually impaired, it is important you ensure spectacles are cleaned and always within reach. Lighting should be bright but without glare, and reading material should be of print size that the older person can read. It may also be helpful to offer the older person the facility of talking newspapers and talking books. In-turned lashes are common in older people and cause irritation of the cornea. Out-turned lashes are also common in older people and cause watery eye (epiphora) (Coni & Webster 1998). You should assess the need for eye care while you are attending to the older person's personal needs.

CARE OF EARS

The ears are also affected by ageing in the older person (Coni & Webster 1998). Sixty per cent of people over 70 are hearing impaired and should be considered for provision of a hearing aid. Wax in the ear becomes more viscous as the person grows older and this tends to blur hearing. It may need to be removed by a registered nurse who is trained and competent to do so. There is a loss of high-frequency hearing and difficulty in hearing when background noise exists. Impaired hearing can lead to poor health. Deafness may be associated with nerve deafness, caused by ageing, drugs or diseases causing compression; or it may be associated with conduction deafness following disease or infection. Hence, a hearing aid may be very important to the older person although it does not give normal hearing. Some sounds are amplified, and it may be difficult to distinguish finer sounds and several voices in conversation. Adaptations to help the older person with hearing difficulty to manage at home include flashing telephones, amplified telephones, vibrating alarm clocks, and a loop system for the TV, as well as the use of subtitles on TV.

When communicating with older people who have impaired hearing it is important you do not shout, but speak clearly and slowly, although not in an exaggerated way. To make lip-reading easier your face should be well lit and your mouth should not be obscured. You should ask the older person if he or she can hear what you are saying. The hearing aid should be properly worn, kept clean, and the battery checked and changed as necessary. If the older person still cannot hear you, communications should be clearly written on paper.

ORAL HYGIENE

Oral hygiene, care of the mouth and teeth, aims to remove plaque and debris to ensure the structures and tissues of the mouth, including dentures, are kept clean, functional, comfortable and free from infection (DOH 2001c). Many older people wear dentures. Sixty-five per cent of people between 65 and 74 have no natural teeth. Eighty-two per cent of people over 75 have no natural teeth (Coni & Webster 1998). A clean and comfortable mouth will improve the appetite and encourage good nutrition and so good health.

THE CARE RELATIONSHIP

In the light of this assessment, you should plan the procedure with the older person and carry it out as agreed together, taking account of any risks such as swallowing, spreading infection and safety. The older person's choice and independence should be encouraged as far as this is realistic and possible. In carrying out the procedure, the older person is the central focus of attention. You should discuss, explain and listen throughout. Sensitivity to the older person's individual needs, and the protection of his or her privacy and dignity are crucial. As a result, a relationship of trust and confidence can be built that will underpin all other aspects of care (DOH 2001a).

When the procedure is completed the older person should be comfortable. This can be checked by asking if his or her needs have been met. All personal items should be left within reach of the older person, including a call bell to give him or her confidence that help is at hand if required. Hygiene needs should be assessed and re-assessed to find out if they have been met effectively, by asking the older person, by observing, and by referring to nursing and medical records (DOH 2001c).

Procedure One   Making or changing the older person's bed with the person still in bed

Care requirements
The older person should feel clean and comfortable in bed. Care should be given by an appropriately trained person.

Care objectives
The bed should be made daily, and sheets changed as necessary, to preserve the older person's comfort and help prevent skin breakdown. The older person's bed-linen/sheets should be changed immediately when soiled, to protect hygiene, comfort and skin integrity. The older person's bed should be stripped and cleaned after discharge or transfer.

Care actions	Rationale
See Symbols 1–5, Chapter 1	
Collect equipment that may be required and place on trolley or clean, cleared surface such as bed extension or a chair: • clean bed-linen • sliding sheet • linen skip • plastic bag for wet and soiled linen • gloves and apron	To promote the older person's dignity, so that you will not have to leave during changing the bed. To be organised in advance in order to be efficient.
Prepare the working area, paying particular attention to the bed height, and position of bed (may need to be moved away from the wall). For ease and economy of movement it is recommended that two people should make the bed, working together in harmony.	To ensure ample working space, to prevent you and any helpers suffering back strain.
Remove unnecessary pillows and place on chair/bed extension.	To make an easier working environment.

Untuck and remove top layers of bedding and fold each piece on bed extension or chair (sheet, blankets, counterpane if used, or duvet) in the order they will be used.	Work in harmony with partner, working from one position to avoid needless journeys up and down the bed.
Ensure that the older person is covered with a sheet or blanket at all times.	Maintain older person's privacy and dignity.
Hold linen away from clothing and without shaking discard dirty linen in linen container. Discard wet and soiled linen as per local policy.	To avoid cross-infection. To separate soiled and wet linen from used linen for laundry treatment.
Change the bottom sheet by asking the older person to roll on to his or her side or use a sliding sheet under the older person to roll them on to their side.	To conform to moving and handling legislation, thus preventing injury to the older person and harm or injury to yourself or any other carers.
Roll up soiled sheet towards the older person's back and unroll clean sheet. Remove sliding sheet if used. Tuck in new sheet edges. Tuck in top edge first, bottom edge next, and side edges last. Mitre the corners by lifting side edges at bottom of bed to form a clean edge, then tuck in. Ensure rough side of sheet on which seams or hems occur is facing away from the bed and the older person.	Use mitres or 'hospital corners' for tidiness and tightness. Use ironed crease in sheet as guide. Keep linens firmly tucked under mattress to prevent wrinkling. If the older person is lying on a pressure relieving mattress do not tuck the sheet in so as not to obstruct air flow. To prevent hems rubbing against the older person.
Ask the older person to roll over on to clean sheet. Or, if necessary, use the sliding sheet to help you roll the older person over. Warn the older person that there will be a lump in the bed.	To conform to moving and handling legislation, thus preventing injury to the older person and yourself or any other carers.
Remove soiled sheet and put in linen container as per local policy.	To prevent cross-infection.
Pull sheet through. Remove sliding sheet if used. Smoothe out creases and tuck in, using 'hospital corners' or mitres.	To remove creases as this may cause pressure on the older person's skin and lead to skin breakdown.

Position the older person for comfort, ensuring you adhere to moving and handling legislation.	To prevent injury or harm to the older person and yourself or any other carers. To maintain the older person's comfort.
Replace pillows, ensuring all pillow-cases are clean/changed as necessary. Dispose of soiled pillow-cases into linen container as per local policy.	To maintain the older person's comfort and prevent cross-infection.
Replace top bed-linen in order, using new linen as required. If using sheets and blankets, rather than duvet and cover, unfold and replace using ironed creases, if present, as a guide to symmetry. Ensure top linen is not restrictive or tight by folding a 7–8 cm pleat over feet. Fold under each blanket at the top, and fold 0.5–1 metre of the top sheet over the blankets so that older person's chest will be covered and edge will be neat.	To ensure the older person's comfort. To prevent restrictions on older person's movement. To allow room for the older person's feet and to prevent pressure that can cause discomfort, skin breakdown and foot-drop. To give the bed a finished appearance.
Adjust bed to required height.	To ensure height of bed facilitates the older person's safety and transfers.

Procedure Two   **Assisting the older person requiring a wash in bed or chair, including care of hands and feet**

Care requirements
The older person requires assistance to wash and dress. Care should be given by an appropriately trained person.

Care objectives
The older person will have washing and dressing requirements met. The older person will feel clean and comfortable.

Care actions	Rationale
See Symbols 1–5, Chapter 1.	
Collect all equipment by the older person's side on clean, clear surface such as trolley or bed-table: • clean bed-linen • blanket/sheet to cover older person • container for used linen • plastic bag for wet and soiled linen • soap or aqueous cream and toiletries of the older person's choice, including comb and/or brush • towel and clean, dry cloths/disposable cloths • clean night-clothes/day-clothes as appropriate • disposable wipes for incontinence • rubbish bag for disposing of debris • washing bowl containing warm water • mouth-care equipment (according to need, see mouth-care procedure) • shaving equipment if needed • nail-care equipment (including nail clippers if nails are long, and cotton buds if nails are dirty) • small mirror • cosmetics if worn • clinical waste bag • gloves and apron	To promote the older person's dignity, in that you will not have to leave during the procedure. To be organised in advance in order to be efficient. The older person's skin tends to dryness owing to reduction in sebaceous excretion, so keep skin moist and avoid irritants. Nails become thicker and harder in the older person. Fabric cloths become colonised with micro-organisms when left damp. Warm, moist areas of the body, such as the axillae, the genitals, anal area, buttocks and groins are heavily colonised with bacteria. Cloths should be changed/discarded after washing these areas. Washing water should be changed when tepid and/or dirty, and after washing genitals, buttocks and anal region. Position mirror so that the older person can see his/her face.

Ask the older person whether they prefer soap or aqueous cream on the face. Using firm and gentle strokes wash, rinse and dry face carefully: eyelids, forehead, cheeks, nose, ears and jaw. Finish with neck. If the older person is willing and able, help the older person to do this himself/herself.	To promote cleanliness and comfort. To maintain independence. Older person's skin tends to dryness owing to reduction in sebaceous excretion, so keep skin moist and avoid irritants.
If required assist with shave, or enable older person to shave themselves. (A woman may require assistance with removal of facial hair if needed.) Keep skin tight if wet shaving, lathering well first to soften skin and help prevent pulling, scraping and cutting skin. Shave in direction of hair growth. Dry carefully. Change water following wet shave.	Men may like to shave daily – use a wet razor or electric razor. There is an increase in facial hair in women. If skin bleeds during shave apply pressure with a swab until bleeding stops.
Place a towel on the bed under the older person's arm which is furthest away from you. Using a new flannel and starting at the hand, work from the hand up the arm and finish at the axilla. If soap used, rinse off the soap in the same manner.	Try not to lean across the older person; use a partner if possible to minimise strain to you and protect the older person's comfort.
Using the towel, dry his/her fingers, hands, arms and axilla. Repeat the procedure with the other arm.	Wet, moist skin will cause soreness and is an ideal place for micro-organisms.
Uncover the older person's chest. Use a flannel to wash the chest, starting at the upper chest and working down to the groin. If soap is used, rinse the soap off carefully.	To make sure the older person is comfortable.
Dry chest with towel and then cover the chest.	Wet, moist skin will cause soreness and is an ideal place for micro-organisms. To maintain the older person's dignity and ensure he/she does not get cold.

Change water if necessary.	To make sure the older person is comfortable and to provide sufficient clean water to rinse off soap, which might otherwise have a drying effect on the skin.
Remove older person's lower clothes including any thrombo-embolic deterrent stockings. Place towel under the furthest leg, cover genitals and nearest leg.	To maintain older person's privacy and dignity. Do not lean across the older person; use partner if possible to wash furthest side to minimise strain to you and protect the older person's comfort.
Using a new cloth/wipe, wash, rinse and dry the uncovered leg from knee up, then wash, rinse and dry from knee to ankle, then using a new wipe/cloth, wash, rinse and dry the foot and between the toes. Elevate the leg by supporting the ankle. If the older person is able to carry out some or all of this, give help as required. Use firm and gentle strokes. Wash and dry the leg nearest you in the same way.	To maintain the older person's comfort. To promote independence.
If the older person is in a chair they may like to put feet in a bowl of water.	To maintain the older person's comfort.
Check toenails; cut them if required and/or clean them. The older person may need to be referred to a podiatrist.	To promote cleanliness and comfort for the older person. Apathy, stiff hips and obesity may mean that toenails are not cut. Unless the older person has very distorted nails, diabetes mellitus or arteriosclerosis nails may be cut with clippers. If they are very hard they may be softened by soaking in warm water for ten minutes. Good light is needed, and only the distal part of the nail protruding beyond the toe needs to be cut. If the older person is diabetic and has areas of numbness in the feet and/or has corns, calluses or veruccas, seek specialist help from a podiatrist.

Change water if necessary.	To promote cleanliness and comfort and prevent infection.
Using a new flannel/wipe, wash and dry genitalia. Wash from the front of the perineal area to the back. In the male older person ensure that the foreskin is repositioned after washing and drying underneath it.	To promote cleanliness and comfort and prevent infection. To prevent inflammation and swelling of the end of the penis.
If the older person is in bed and is unable to roll on to his or her side independently, you will need another carer to assist washing his/her back.	To minimise strain to you and protect the older person's comfort.
With two carers, one either side of the bed, roll the older person on to his/her side and support them. Sheets can also be changed as per previous instructions at the same time.	To minimise strain to you and protect the older person's comfort. To save time.
Place a towel alongside the older person's back to prevent the sheets/mattress getting wet.	To protect the older person's comfort.
If the older person is sitting in a chair, ask them to lean forward in order for you to wash their back.	To promote cleanliness and comfort.
Wash and dry the older person's back, starting at the shoulders and working down towards the bottom.	To promote cleanliness and comfort.
Using new wipe/flannel, wash and dry the older person's buttocks and anal area.	To promote cleanliness and comfort. To prevent infection.
If the older person is in a chair, help them to stand and assist in washing and drying buttocks and anal area. Depending on how steady the older person is on their feet you may need another carer to assist.	To promote cleanliness and comfort. To minimise strain to you and protect the older person's comfort.

Throughout the wash check and observe skin integrity over bony prominences for redness, discoloration or damage, and for physical condition: ear, occiput, shoulder blades, spine, elbow, inside knee, heel and ankle, sacrum, iliac crest, hip.	To observe for changes and areas of pressure prone to develop into pressure ulcers.
Pay particular attention to skin folds.	Skin folds may become moist with micro-organisms.
Assist older person to put on clothes/ nightwear as appropriate. If older person has a weak side, or has an infusion, put clothes on affected side first. Position the older person for comfort. Replace top layers of bedclothes if in bed. Assist older person to put on slippers/shoes and blanket, if required, if in chair, and elevate legs and feet if necessary. Offer mouth care according to mouth-care procedure. Help the older person to comb hair. Help the older person to apply cosmetics and/or nail varnish if required.	To promote cleanliness and comfort. For ease of movement. To reduce risk of pressure ulcers. To maintain independence. To maintain cleanliness.

Procedure Three   Assisting the older person to wash in the bath or shower, including care of hands and feet

Care requirements
The older person requires assistance to bathe or shower. Care should be given by an appropriately trained person.

Care objectives
The older person will be enabled to bathe or shower. The older person will feel comfortable.

Care actions	Rationale
See Symbols 1–5, Chapter 1.	
Make sure there are no draughts in bath or shower room and that the room is warm. Ensure bath or shower is clean.	To maintain the older person's comfort and dignity. To prevent infection.
Collect all equipment in bath/shower room: • soap or aqueous cream and toiletries of the older person's choice, including comb and/or brush • towel and clean, dry cloths/disposable cloths • clean day-clothes as appropriate • mouth-care equipment • shaving equipment if needed • nail-care equipment (including cotton buds if nails are dirty, or nail clippers if nails are long) • cosmetics if used • small mirror • gloves and apron • clinical waste bag	To promote the older person's dignity, in that you will not have to leave during the procedure. To be organised in advance in order to be efficient. The older person's skin tends to dryness greasy owing to reduction in sebaceous excretion, so keep skin moist and avoid irritants. Nails become thicker and harder in the older person, and there is an increase in facial hair in women. Fabric cloths become colonised with micro-organisms when left damp. Warm, moist areas of the body, such as the axillae, the genitals, anal area, buttocks and groin are heavily colonised with bacteria. Cloths should be changed/discarded after washing these areas.

If using bath, half fill the bath with water, running the cold water first and then the hot. Stir the water up and use the elbow to check the bath water is the appropriate temperature for the older person. Ensure bath/shower mat is available if required.	To ensure the water is at the correct temperature. To safeguard the older person from falling.
If the older person is able to bath/shower unaided, ensure clothes and equipment are in reach. Ensure call bell is within reach or that they are able to call for attention if at home. Close the door but do not lock it. Ensure notice is available to show room is occupied if in hospital/care home.	To allow for the older person's privacy and dignity and to ensure safety and comfort.
If the older person requires assistance, help to remove clothes. If the older person has an affected side, or has an infusion, remove clothes from unaffected side first. Cover the older person with towels.	To allow for the older person's privacy and dignity and to ensure safety and comfort.
Position bath hoist, and explain and demonstrate how it works. Help the older person into hoist, ensuring he/she feels safe and comfortable. Depending on the older person's ability to move, you may need assistance of another carer. Keep non-slip shoes/slippers on while assisting the older person to transfer. Raise the hoist and lower the older person into bath. Evaluate the older person's comfort and safety throughout.	To allow for the older person's privacy and dignity and to make sure of safety and comfort. To minimise strain to you and protect the older person's comfort.
Help the older person to wash according to procedure for the older person requiring assistance with personal hygiene.	To promote cleanliness and comfort.
Use towel/s to cover the older person. Raise the hoist and help the older person out of bath and on to chair. Assist the older person to dry, pay particular attention to skin folds.	To maintain the older person's comfort. To promote independence. Skin folds may become moist with micro-organisms.

Throughout the wash check and observe skin integrity over bony prominences for redness, discoloration or damage and for physical condition: ear, occiput, shoulder blades, spine, elbow, inside knee, heel and ankle, sacrum, iliac crest, hip.	To observe for changes and areas of pressure prone to develop into pressure ulcers.
Check toenails, if required clean the nails and/or cut them. The older person may need to be referred to a podiatrist.	To promote cleanliness and comfort for the older person. Apathy, stiff hips and obesity may mean that toenails are not cut. Unless the older person has very distorted nails, diabetes mellitus or arteriosclerosis nails may be cut with clippers. If they are very hard they may be softened by soaking in warm water for ten minutes. Good light is needed, and only the distal part of the nail protruding beyond the toe needs to be cut.
Check fingernails, trim and/or clean if required.	To promote cleanliness and comfort.
If using shower, assist the older person to transfer to shower chair (rather than hoist) and follow above instructions.	To promote cleanliness and comfort. To maintain older person's safety.
Help with shave, removal of facial hair, mouth care and hair care as required, giving assistance as necessary.	To promote cleanliness and comfort. To promote the older person's independence.
Assist the older person to put on clothes/nightware as appropriate. If older person has a weak side, or has an infusion, put clothes on affected side first. Position the older person for comfort. Replace top layers of bedclothes if in bed. Assist older person to put on slippers/shoes and blanket, if required, if in chair, and elevate legs and feet if necessary. Help the older person to apply cosmetics and/or nail varnish if required.	To promote cleanliness and comfort. For ease of movement. To reduce risk of pressure ulcers. To maintain independence. To maintain cleanliness.

Procedure Four   Assisting the bed-bound older person to wash his or her hair

Care requirements
The older person is in bed and requires help to wash hair and is unable to sit in a chair. Care should be given by an appropriately trained person.

Care objectives
The older person will be enabled to wash hair. The older person's hair will feel clean and comfortable.

Care actions	Rationale
See Symbols 1–5, Chapter 1.	
Collect all equipment by bedside: • shampoo of the older person's choice, comb and/or brush • 2 towels • 2 washing bowls • large jug • bedfast rinser instead of washing bowl (if available) • waterproof pad • hairdryer • mirror • gloves and apron	To promote the older person's dignity, so that you will not have to leave during the procedure. To be organised in order to be efficient.
Adjust bed height if possible. Pull bed away from wall and remove bed-head/backrest. Use flat bedhead or table behind bed. Cover with waterproof pad and towel and place bedfast rinser or second bowl on top. If using bedfast rinser, place bowl on floor to receive rinsed water.	To make space and prepare for procedure. To avoid back strain or injury to yourself.
Check scalp for irritation before beginning procedure. Position the older person on his/her back with head overhanging mattress. Remove or push back upper clothing. Cover top half of body with towel.	The older person's scalp may be irritated because skin tends to be thin and hair is brittle. To enable the older person to protect dignity and keep as comfortable and dry as possible.

Fill bowl with warm water. Use elbow to test.	To ensure the water is at the correct temperature.
Using the jug and water from the bowl carefully wet the older person's hair and allow water to fall on to bedfast rinser if used, or second bowl. Use shampoo to wash hair. Rinse, and repeat if necessary. Apply conditioner and rinse if required.	To ensure hair is clean and that the older person is comfortable throughout procedure.
Position mirror so that the older person can see his/her face and hair. Towel the hair dry and dry hair with hairdryer if required. Comb the hair. Position for comfort.	To promote comfort.

Procedure Five   Assisting the older person with cleansing of the mouth, including care of dentures

Care requirements
The older person needs assistance to maintain integrity and hygiene of mouth, gums, teeth, tongue and lips. Care should be given by an appropriately trained person.

Care objectives
To keep the mucosa and lips clean, pink, soft, moist and intact and to prevent infection. To remove debris and dental plaque without damaging the gingiva. To alleviate discomfort, promote healing, reduce infection, enhance oral intake (if able to swallow) and freshen the mouth. To assess frequency and method of oral hygiene to be used. The older person will feel comfortable.

Care actions	Rationale
See Symbols 1–5, Chapter 1.	
Prepare equipment: • small mirror for the older person • clinically clean tray • good light source, spatula • receiver/small bowl, mouthwash tablets, water, saline • plastic beaker • tube of yellow paraffin • swab for removal of dentures • sponge swabs/foam sticks • soft toothbrush and/or the older person's own toothbrush • toothpaste • labelled denture container and lid • towel and paper tissues • gloves and apron • clinical waste bag	To promote the older person's dignity so that you will not have to leave during the procedure. To be organised in order to be efficient. Many older people wear dentures they are not happy with because they are ill-fitting, since gums recede with age. Many choose not to wear them. Comfortable dentures promote nutrition. Denture containers should be labelled to avoid loss of dentures. Toothbrush should be washed and left to dry after use to avoid growth of micro-organisms. Toothbrushes should be replaced every 6–12 weeks to be effective. Position mirror so the older person can see his/her face.

Help the older person to sit in a comfortable position. If possible, position the older person next to a wash basin. Otherwise, the older person should sit in an upright position either in a chair or bed. If there are reasons why the older person is unable to sit upright, or is unconscious, help them on to their side, cover the pillow with a waterproof cover and a towel. Depending on the older person's ability to move, you may need the assistance of another carer. Protect the older person's clothing with a towel.	To protect the older person's dignity. To avoid back strain of carer. It is preferable for the older person to sit upright for access to mouth and to prevent excess fluid running down throat or face. If the older person is unable to sit up, the older person should be positioned on his/her side, so that excess fluid drains out of mouth.
Ask the older person to remove dentures, or, if unable, remove them by using a swab. Place in a denture pot with clean water.	Dentures should be removed carefully, to reduce contact with saliva, and to enable inspection of mouth.
Assess the older person's mouth. Note any ulcers, sores, food debris, colour and furring of tongue.	Restricted fluid intake, mouth-breathing or oxygen therapy will reduce production of saliva and dry oral mucosa. Reduced physical dexterity and/or mental competence limit the older person's ability to maintain own oral hygiene. Some antibiotics produce discoloration or damage and furring of tongue.
Using a small toothbrush and toothpaste, brush the older person's natural teeth, tongue and gums. Brush inner and outer aspects with firm individual strokes directed towards gums.	To remove adherent materials from the teeth, tongue and gum surfaces. Brushing stimulates gingival tissues to maintain tone, prevents circulatory stasis and reduces pathogenic organisms.
Give a beaker of water or mouthwash, diluted as recommended, to the older person to rinse mouth vigorously and void into receiver or small bowl. Paper tissues should be at hand.	Rinsing removes loosened debris and freshens mouth. Mouth cleansers should be used with caution. Inappropriate dilution and long-term use can damage oral mucosa.

If the older person is unable to rinse and void mouth, use soft moistened toothbrush to clean teeth and sponge swabs moistened in saline, water or mouthwash liquid, diluted appropriately, to wipe gums and oral mucosa. Rotate sponge swabs to utilise all the surface. Gentle suction may be used to remove excess secretions.	Discard remaining mouthwash to prevent risk of contamination. Sponge swabs produce less friction than toothbrushes but do not clean so well.
If the older person has thick mucus, sodium bicarbonate solution may be used before rinsing mouth with saline or water.	This will dissolve the mucus.
Only if appropriate, and the person is able to swallow, you may give soda water, fresh fruit, and ice cubes to moisten the mouth.	If older person can swallow, this will moisten mouth, stimulate production of saliva and aid comfort.
If lips are dry, lubricate with soft yellow paraffin. Apply with gloved finger or gauze swab.	To promote comfort and alleviate dryness.
Clean dentures with denture paste or soap and water, or soak in chlorhexidine solution for ten minutes. Rinse well. Inspect for cracks. Return to older person's mouth or, if not in use, store in cold water in named denture container with lid. Use tissue to wipe any moisture from lips.	To make sure the older person is comfortable and to reduce risk of infection. Soak in chlorhexidine solution if oral candida is present. Some denture cleaners may have an abrasive effect on denture surfaces. This attracts plaque and encourages bacterial growth.

Procedure Six   Assisting the older person requiring eye care

Care requirements
The older person has debris on eyelids and/or eyelashes. Care should be given by an appropriately trained person.

Care objectives
The risk of infection will be reduced. The debris will be removed. The older person will feel comfortable.

Care actions	Rationale
See Symbols 1–5, Chapter 1.	
Prepare equipment on clean bed table: • sterilised gauze/low-linting swabs • sterile water/normal saline • gallipot or small sterilised receiver or small sterilised bowl • clean, clear area on bed-table/or clean trolley • small mirror • gloves and apron • clinical waste bag	To promote the older person's dignity, so that you will not have to leave during the procedure. To be organised in order to be efficient. Although this is not a sterile procedure, it is advisable to use materials and equipment that are as free from contamination as possible to reduce the risk of introducing infection. Use low-linting swabs to avoid fibres becoming detached into eyes. Position mirror so that older person can see his/her face.
The older person can sit or lie, with their head tilted backwards and well supported. Make sure there is an adequate light source. Do not dazzle the older person.	To protect the older person's dignity and provide comfort. To enable maximum observation of the eyes without causing the older person harm or discomfort.
You should adjust bed height to comfortable working height if possible, and stand at the same side of the older person as the eye to be cleansed.	To provide you with good access to the eye and avoid back strain.

Always treat the unaffected eye first.	To avoid cross-infection.
Eyes should be closed when lids are bathed.	To avoid damage to cornea.
Moisten swab slightly, ask the older person to look up and swab lower lid from nasal corner outwards.	If swab is too wet the solution will run down the older person's cheek, increasing the risk of cross-infection and causing discomfort. Swabbing from nasal corner outwards avoids the risk of nasal discharge into lachrymal punctum, or even across bridge of nose into other eye.
Make sure that edge of swab is not above the lid margin.	To avoid touching sensitive cornea.
Use a new swab each time, repeating the procedure until all discharge has been removed.	To reduce the risk of infection.
Swab the upper lid by slightly everting the lid margin and asking the older person to look down. Swab from the nasal corner outwards and use a new swab each time until all discharge has been removed. Repeat if necessary.	To remove foreign material from eye. To reduce the risk of infection.

3   Care for the older person requiring assistance with movement

VICKY MACARTHUR

This chapter discusses the knowledge and skills you will need to help the older person safely with movement. This aspect of care is often referred to as 'moving and handling' or 'manual handling', and all those caring for older persons in a 'professional' capacity are required by law to have received training in this aspect of care, including annual updates of this training. The legal background can be found in the moving and handling section of this book (pp. 19–20), and you should refer to this before continuing.

As a carer, one of your primary aims should always be to safeguard the health and well-being of the older person. Much of the material in this chapter will help you to achieve this aim during assistance with movement. However, this chapter will also be concerned with your own health and well-being.

According to the Health and Safety Executive (2005) one in five of those reporting illnesses at work suffer from back pain, and manual handling is a major cause of back injury. In the period between 1996 and 2001 over 61 000 workers in the health service suffered a work-related injury, the majority of those (over 50 per cent) that resulted in absences longer than three days were due to manual handling. It was also found that 60 per cent of all manual handling accidents reported in the NHS involve patient handling, suggesting that staff working with patients are most at risk. Department of Health statistics have estimated that back pain is costing the NHS £481 million each year (NHS Plus 2006a). While this financial cost is serious at a time when the NHS seems to be shorter of money than ever before, the personal cost can be equally devastating. It is estimated that approximately 3600 nurses are forced to retire each year because of back problems (NHS Plus 2006b), and chronic pain restricts their quality of life.

So, in this chapter we will be considering your own needs in equal measure to those of the older person, in order to ensure that all those involved in manual handling do so safely with as small a risk of injury as is possible.

ASSISTING THE OLDER PERSON TO MOVE

The figures above suggest that manual handling of an older person is a particularly high-risk activity. When you think about your own practice you may be able to identify why this is. Compare, for example, moving a heavy object such as a wardrobe, with moving a person. At first it may seem that the wardrobe, which is likely to be much heavier than the older person, should be more risky and difficult to move. But we would never dream of attempting to move a wardrobe on our own. A wardrobe can be repositioned to make it easier to carry – for example by tipping it on to its side. A wardrobe will not become frightened and grab out at rails or handlers, will not struggle, have 'off days' or have legs that may suddenly give way. We can leave the wardrobe where it is until we have the time, help or right equipment to move it safely. Moving the older person can be much more complicated. The trickiest thing about moving the older person is that he or she does not have 'handles'. This is why we should not be tempted to move the older person using methods that are now considered to be unsafe – for example by using the arms as handles. See pp. 76–9 for more information about unsafe techniques.

AGE-RELATED CHANGES

Moving and handling carries more risk for the older person than for a younger person, because of age-related changes in the body.

MUSCULOSKELETAL CHANGES

Observation of the older person will give clues as to the variety of musculoskeletal changes that occur with age – for example, enlarged joints, stooping, decreased height and flabby muscles (Eliopoulos 2001). Bones undergo changes in texture, degree of calcification and shape, restricting movement and leaving the older person at serious risk of fractures. These fractures often occur in the spinal bones (vertebrae) and this, along with thinning of the vertebral disks and shortening of the vertebrae, results in the reduced height and stooping (kyphosis) mentioned above (Thibodeau & Patton 2004). Muscles become flabby (atrophied) with decreased muscle mass, strength and movement, resulting in slower movement and weakness (Eliopoulos 2001).

During help with movement, you will need to be aware of these changes and allow for slower movement and the possibility of leg and arm weakness. Techniques that put undue stress on the older person's joints, for example the drag lift, should be avoided to prevent damage to muscle and bones in the vulnerable shoulder joint.

SENSORY ORGANS

The sense organs all show a gradual decline with age. Vision starts to deteriorate from the age of 40–45 onwards and many older people require glasses to correct long-sightedness (Thibodeau & Patton 2004). Peripheral vision can be affected and light perception altered, so that the older person may require more light to see properly. Depth perception can change, making it difficult for the older person to judge the height of kerbs and steps. In a review of the literature Moore and Miller (2003) found that poor vision was associated with falls resulting in fractures and dislocations, showing the effects that poor vision has on mobility. Cataracts, which cause the lens of the eye to become cloudy, are a common age-related change which impairs vision.

In many older people hearing can be affected by changes in the inner ear resulting in the inability to hear certain frequencies, initially high-frequency sounds. This can make it particularly difficult to hear speech when there is much background noise (Strawbridge et al. 2000). Speech can sound distorted as high-pitched sounds (consonants such as s, sh, f, ph, ch) are not well heard (Eliopoulos 2001). Changes in the inner ear can also affect balance, which in turn will increase risks during walking.

During assistance with movement you will need to be aware that the older person may not be able to see as well as you in the same lighted conditions and may need to be given more time when tackling steps and kerbs. In addition, the older person may not be aware of surrounding activity because of reduced peripheral vision. Finally, the older person may not be able to hear well enough to participate in manoeuvres by following instructions. However, talking more loudly may not be helpful as this produces a higher-pitched sound which exacerbates the problem and can cause discomfort. When you give instructions you should try to speak clearly and make sure your face can be seen by the person to be moved.

INTEGUMENTARY SYSTEM (SKIN)

Skin elasticity is reduced as a result of cellular changes. As the skin becomes less elastic it can also become dry and fragile with less subcutaneous fat (Thibodeau & Patton 2004). During assistance with movement, manoeuvres that involve handling the limbs should be avoided or performed carefully to prevent tearing the older person's fragile skin. With age-related slowing of wound healing, these tears can become a serious problem since they can be slow to heal, and may lead to chronic wounds. Handling equipment such as slings may be experienced as more uncomfortable as the lack of subcutaneous fat reduces 'padding' around bony areas. Choosing equipment and accessories carefully may help to avoid this problem and make the experience more positive and more likely to be consented to in future.

BRAIN AND NERVOUS SYSTEM

The function of nerve cells decreases with age because these cells are not continually replaced by the body as other cells are. Transmission of signals by the nerves is slower with age, resulting in slower reactions to stimuli such as pain. Some functions in the brain are affected with age, such as learning and memory (Bond, Coleman & Pearce 1999). It should be remembered however that cognitive decline is not a part of normal ageing and it should not be assumed that the older person will suffer from some sort of dementia, as in fact only 2–3 per cent of the population over 65 years do. This proportion increases with age (Bond, Coleman & Pearce 1999). During assistance with movement, you should be prepared to spend a little longer allowing the older person to react to instructions and requests. Instructions about how to participate in manoeuvres should be repeated as frequently as needed to allow for memory problems, if they exist.

The older person is, by virtue of having lived so long, more likely to have other health conditions that may affect these systems such as osteo-arthritis affecting the joints, glaucoma affecting the vision, stroke (cerebro-vascular incidents) affecting their cognitive and physical ability. This should be remembered when helping the older person with movement.

All these factors should be included in the risk assessment, where the 'load' – the older person – is considered.

ASSISTED MOVEMENT TECHNIQUES

Before you start any manual handling tasks remember AARR! This stands for Avoid, Assess, Reduce and Review (Centaur 1999). We have considered the 'Assess' and 'Review' parts of this in an earlier section (pp. 20–1). Familiarise yourself with this before continuing. In this chapter we will be looking at the 'Avoid' and 'Reduce' parts, that is, avoiding unnecessary manual handling in the first place, and reducing the risks to you and the older person by using better techniques and/or equipment.

PROMOTING INDEPENDENCE

Before undertaking any assisted movement think: 'Is it necessary for me to manually assist this person, or could he or she do it himself/herself given more time or the right equipment?' There are two benefits from approaching manual handling tasks in this way. Firstly, all manual handling carries risk. No matter how good your technique or how technological the equipment, you cannot eliminate risk altogether. Just by stooping down to help somebody with his or her shoes, means that you are risking injury to your back. Therefore, the less manual handling you do the less risk of injury. If you can enable the older person to move himself/herself with verbal assistance or equipment, so much the better. Secondly, unnecessary manual handling, where the older person could move himself/herself, is not therapeutic. That is, by doing *for* the older person, you prevent them developing the ability to do it for themselves. Rehabilitation is a key aim of care. By helping the older person to help himself or herself you are moving towards this aim. As we saw in the Introduction, much of the literature states that muscle weakness associated with age can be prevented or reversed to some extent by promoting the older person's mobility (Bond, Coleman & Pearce 1999; Eliopoulos 2001).

There are many pieces of equipment that can be used to promote independence. Some examples are given below. More information about aids to promote independence can be gained from an occupational therapist, district nurse or back-care adviser.

Beds

The hospital bed is an under-valued piece of manual handling equipment! Many areas now have profiling beds which have three or four moving sections in the base. They are electrically operated via a hand control and can raise the person into a sitting position or raise the legs. This eliminates the need for you to do any of these things manually.

Where possible the older person to be moved should be told how to use the bed for themselves. Where you need to operate the bed for the older person, it is essential that you know how to use the control properly to avoid reducing the confidence the older person has in your ability to care for them. You should know how to operate the bed in an emergency situation.

It is possible for the older person to obtain a hospital bed in their own home. However, the majority of older people living at home will not have specially adapted beds and therefore you or other carers are at greater risk from the limitations that domestic beds present. For example, beds may be very low, causing you to stoop while helping with movement. If you are assisting the older person in a double bed to move you are in danger of over-reaching, because the 'load' (the older person) is too far away from your centre of gravity.

Being aware of these risk factors allows you to build them in to the risk assessment and reduce these risks as far as is possible. For example, when helping the older person in a low bed, remembering to kneel down to carry out manoeuvres will avoid the risk of stooping. When assisting with movement in a double bed, you may consider the best solution to be kneeling on the bed in order to get closer to the 'load'. This is no longer considered good practice, and indeed should not be necessary in hospital. Importantly it can result in cross-infection between patients, as discussed below.

Rope ladders

This is a simple piece of equipment that attaches to the bottom of any bed in hospital or home which allows the older person with sufficient upper arm strength to sit up in bed from a lying position. The plastic rungs of the ladder are gripped, and using a 'hand-over-hand' movement the older person gradually pulls himself/herself up into a sitting position (Diagram 1).

Hand blocks

These blocks can be used singly or in pairs. They are used to aid independent movement in bed and will allow the older person to help during movement. The blocks are placed on either side of the older person, who, by pushing down on them, can raise himself/herself from the bed to relieve pressure or move up the bed (Diagram 2).

Bed levers

This is a grab rail that is secured under the mattress and enables the older person to turn over in bed unassisted, or to help during manual handling manoeuvres (Diagram 3).

Lifting pole

Also known as a 'monkey pole', this can be attached to the bed, be wall-fixed or free standing and is used by the older person with good upper body strength to help when sitting up in bed (Diagram 4).

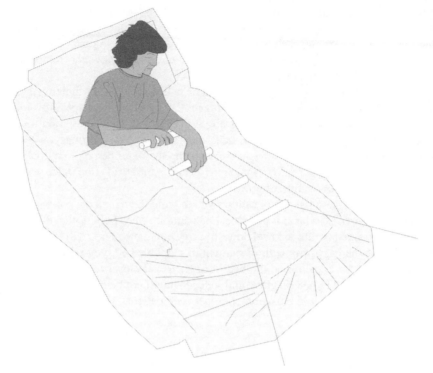

Diagram 1   Rope ladder.

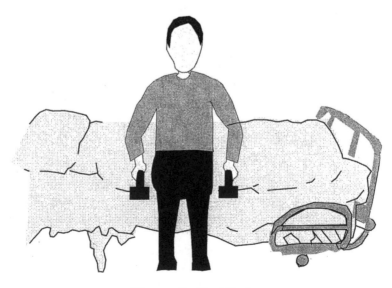

Diagram 2   Hand blocks.

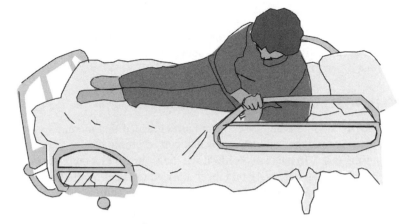

Diagram 3 Bed levers.

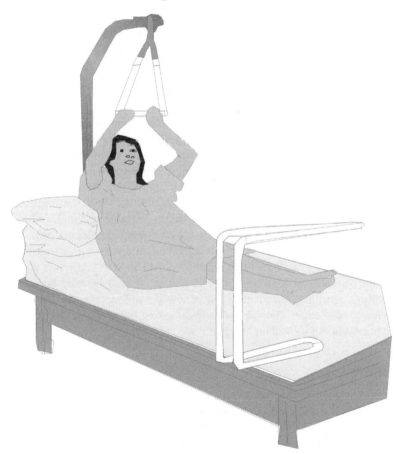

Diagram 4 Lifting pole.

Small sliding sheet

When combined with hand blocks, a lifting pole or bed lever, a small sliding sheet (see below) can reduce friction enough for the older person with less upper arm strength to move himself/herself in bed.

WHEN MANUAL ASSISTANCE IS NEEDED

When the moving and handling assessment has confirmed that manual assistance is necessary, there are recognised techniques that can be employed for many common manual handling tasks. In the cases below it will be assumed that there are two carers available. In many areas carers are no longer allowed to kneel on the bed as this can result in cross-infection from skin cells picked up on the uniform or clothing and transferred to another person's bed. Therefore all techniques described will avoid the handler kneeling on the bed. There are many variations of the techniques below and only the most basic manoeuvres will be described. More information can be found in *The Guide to the Handling of People* (Smith 2005).

The equipment used in these techniques is readily available and should form part of the resources available to you in a clinical area, or via a GP surgery or district nursing team. The two items used below are described.

Sliding sheets

These are made from strong nylon material that has been treated with silicone to enable friction-free movements. There are various types and sizes but they fall into two categories: roller glides and flat sheets. Roller glides are lengths of this material sewn in a long roller band, which is wide enough for the older person to lie on. They may also have webbing handles along the edges. Care should be taken to ensure that the sliding surfaces of the roller are on the inside of the roller before using, as some of these sheets have one non-slide surface. Flat sheets are large rectangles of the same material with hemmed edges. They may also have webbing handles on them. They are used in pairs for moving the older person in the bed, or singly with a transfer board. In the latter case they should be fitted with extended straps to allow safe movement. They are all washable at high temperatures and should not be used between older people without washing. Alternatively, it is now possible to buy 'disposable' slide sheets which are cheaper, though not as long-lasting but designed to be discarded after the person being moved no longer has a need for them.

Handling belts

These are large often padded belts that are worn by the older person and provide the carer with something to hold while helping the older person to mobilise. Handling belts usually have several webbing loops around the circumference of the belt giving alternative holding points, and are fastened by a buckle and/or Velcro. They can also be used, unbuckled, as a sling for lifting legs.

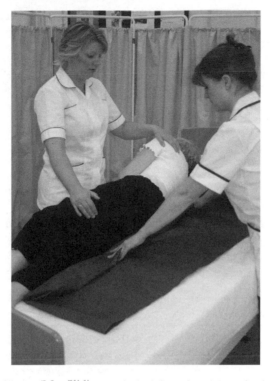

Figure 3.1   Sliding up the bed: Inserting sliding sheet.

Procedure Seven   Assisting the older person to move up the bed

Care requirements
The older person has slipped down the bed, having been in a semi-recumbent position supported by pillows or a backrest and is unable to move himself/herself up the bed. Care should be given by an appropriately trained person.

Care objectives
The older person will be assisted back to a semi-recumbent position. The older person will be comfortable. This is most easily achieved in two stages, first sliding the person to be moved up the bed in a lying position and then sitting him/her forward.

Care actions	Rationale
See Symbols 1–5, Chapter 1.	
Collect a sliding sheet.	If the older person is too large or heavy for two staff to use a sliding sheet, then you will need to use a hoist. A one-way sliding sheet may help in preventing the older person slipping down the bed in the first place, as will raising the knees on a profiling bed.
The backrest is lowered and/or pillows are removed so that the older person to be moved is lying flat.	This allows for sliding the older person up the bed.
You and another carer stand on either side of the older person's bed. Where possible, the bed should be at hip height of the shortest carer.	This avoids the need for stooping, thus reducing the risk of injury. The taller carer should bend at the knees to avoid stooping.
Log-roll the older person and insert the slide sheet. Ensure the sliding sheet extends from the top of the head to the feet – if it does not, insert a small sliding sheet under the feet (Figure 3.1).	Any contact between the older person and the bed will increase the effort required to move them and may damage the skin of the older person as they are moved.

Place a pillow up against the head of the bed.	This prevents banging the older person's head on the headboard as you may be stronger than you think!
Each carer is required to stand facing the foot of the bed – diagonally towards the opposite corner (Figure 3.2).	This avoids any twisting during the manoeuvre which would increase the risk of injury.
Each carer grips the upper layer of the sliding sheet, the nearest hand to the older person to be moved at the older person's shoulder level, the other hand at hip level (Figure 3.3).	Again, this prevents twisting.
Carers should have an L-shaped base with their weight on the front foot.	This increases the carers' stability.
On the agreed command from the designated leader, the carers transfer their weight to their back foot and without bending their arms too much bring the older person back with them on the sliding sheet.	This means that the carers use their body weight to move the older person rather than the physical effort of pulling. This helps to avoid upper back stress.
Repeat if necessary rather than attempting it in one go.	Moving a distance may result in twisting.

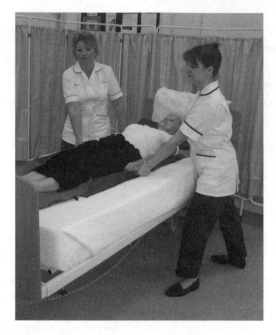

Figure 3.2   Sliding up the bed: starting position.

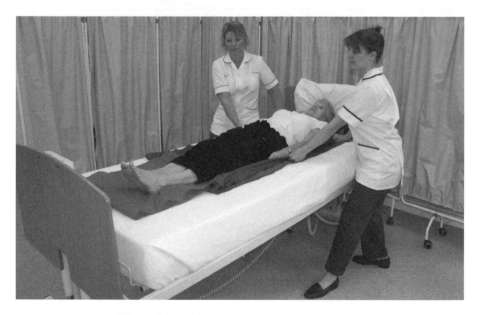

Figure 3.3   Sliding up the bed: finishing position.

Procedure Eight   Assisting the older person to move from a lying to a sitting position

Care requirements
The older person wishes to be sat up, having been lying flat or slumped, and requires assistance. The older person is lying flat or is semi-recumbent and needs to sit forward to allow for repositioning of pillows, insertion of a sling or personal hygiene needs. Care should be given by an appropriately trained person.

Care objectives
To help the older person into a sitting position supported by a backrest or pillow. The older person will be comfortable.

Care actions	Rationale
See Symbols 1–5, Chapter 1.	
Consider whether it is necessary to manually assist the older person. Equipment could include: • rope ladder or lifting pole so the older person can participate or perform the move independently • handling slings or netting if head support needed; same technique • profiling bed • pillow lift or sit-u-up, e.g. Mangar equipment.	The task can be done more safely using equipment that is easy to purchase, and therefore this technique should be done on a short-term basis only. An appropriate piece of equipment should be obtained as soon as possible.
Two carers stand facing the older person, on either side of the bed. The bed is at hip height for the shortest carer.	This avoids the need for stooping, thus reducing the risk of injury. The taller person should bend at the knees.
Each carer places the hand that is nearest the older person over the top of the shoulder, sliding it down the back to cover the shoulder blade (scapula) (Figure 3.4).	Using the nearest hand avoids twisting during the manoeuvre.

Insert the other hand under the side of the older person at a right angle to the first hand (along where the bra would be on a female). Carers are in a slightly forward-leaning posture with an L-shaped base with weight on the front foot (Figure 3.4).	This increases the carers' stability.
Carers raise their heads before starting the manoeuvre (to get the spine in line) and, on an agreed command from the identified leader, transfer weight to the back foot.	Raising the head puts the spine in line ready for the manoeuvre. The agreed command (e.g. 'ready, steady, sit') helps to ensure carers make an equal effort at the same time and the effort is shared.
Without bending the arms, bring the older person into a sitting position as you step back (Figure 3.5).	This means that the carers use their body weight to move the older person, rather than physical effort of pulling. This helps to avoid upper-back stress.

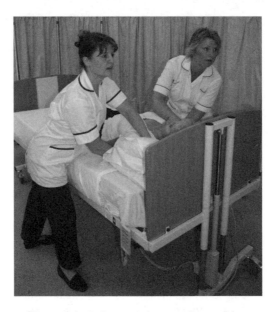

Figure 3.4 Lying to sitting: starting position.

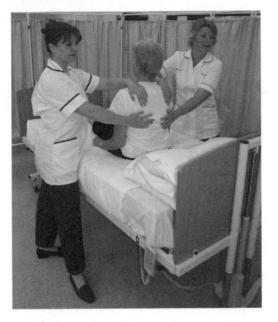

Figure 3.5   Lying to sitting: finishing position.

Procedure Nine   **Assisting the older person with a lateral transfer while they are in a lying position**

Care requirements
The older person needs to be moved from one flat service to another, for example trolley to bed, bed to trolley or bed to bed. Care should be given by an appropriately trained person.

Care objectives
The older person is to be helped to transfer from one flat surface to another. The older person will be comfortable.

Care actions	Rationale
See Symbols 1–5, Chapter 1.	
Gather equipment required: • at least three appropriately trained carers • a hard transfer board, e.g. pat slide • extended strap sliding sheet	Alternatives: roller glide or hoisting
Two carers log-roll the older person and insert the sliding sheet underneath him/her, slippy side down.	Sliding sheet will be in contact with the transfer board placed underneath.
The older person is rolled on to his/her side and supported by one or two carers. Two carers position the transfer board under the older person so that he/she is lying on about one third of the width of the board (Figure 3.6). Roll the older person on to their back	The transfer board will act as a 'bridge' between the two surfaces.
The other carers move the receiving bed/trolley next to the bed; if possible it should be slightly lower than the flat surface the older person is currently on. Ensure brakes are applied to bed/trolley.	A lower receiving surface means gravity will assist the movement, reducing effort.
The extended straps are put over the receiving bed/trolley.	Extended straps mean that it is not necessary for carers to climb on to the receiving bed to reach the sliding sheet.

The two carers position themselves on the far side of the receiving bed/trolley and take a strap each (Figure 3.7). The other carer remains on the opposite side of the bed/trolley to support the older person.	Having two carers ensures the effort is shared and helps to keep the older person straight as they move. Reassurance from an extra carer helps to calm the older person being moved.
With an L-shaped base and their weight on the front foot, on command the two carers transfer their weight on to the back foot and bring the older person on the sliding sheet over on to the receiving bed/trolley (Figure 3.8).	This means that the carers use their body weight to move the person, rather than the physical effort of pulling. This helps to avoid upper-back stress. An L-shaped base increases stability.
The sliding sheet may be placed underneath bed-linen to transfer this with the person to be moved if necessary. Bed-sheets must not be used in place of a sliding sheet.	A bed-sheet is not a recognised piece of handling equipment and does not therefore comply with the legislation.

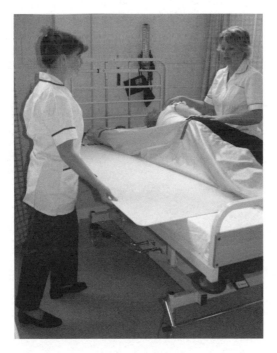

Figure 3.6 Lateral transfer: inserting transfer board.

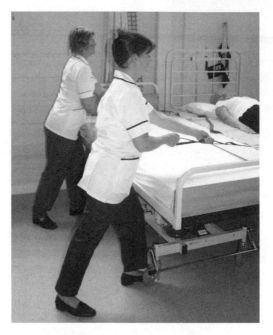

Figure 3.7   Starting position.

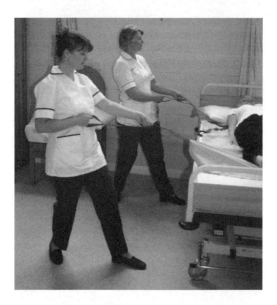

Figure 3.8   Finishing position.

Procedure Ten   Assisting the older person to sit back in the chair

Care requirements
The older person has been sitting in an armchair for some time and has slipped into a slumped position. He/she is unable to move back because of reduced upper-arm strength. Care should be given by an appropriately trained person.

Care objectives
To help the older person back in the chair into a safer and more comfortable position. The older person will be comfortable.

Care actions	Rationale
See Symbols 1–5, Chapter 1.	
Ensure that the older person's feet are placed flat on the floor in front of them. He/she should be helped to put on shoes or slippers, if they have not already got them on.	To prevent the older person slipping to the floor. Shoes help to provide grip.
	This technique works best when the older person is clothed and is sitting on a plastic-covered chair. Two carers may be needed for this technique.
	Sliding sheets should not be used. One-way sliding sheets may help prevent the person slipping in the chair in the first place and will assist with this technique. A hoist will have to be used where this technique is not possible owing to the nature of the furniture or condition of the person to be moved.
Using the scapula grip as described in Procedure Eight, the older person is helped to sit forwards in the chair.	This replaces any drag lift, which is considered unsafe.

If the older person is unable to maintain this position you will require another carer to support them in this position.	
You can then kneel in front of the older person on one or two knees and place a pillow on the front part of the legs of the older person (Figure 3.9).	Kneeling prevents stooping and reduces the risk of injury to the carer. Care should be taken when considering this technique with an older person who is likely to hit out, or a person who has knee or hip injuries.
On an agreed command, the older person is encouraged to use his/her arms on the arms of the chair to take as much weight as he/she is able (if any) while you gently but firmly push against their knees through the pillow. The older person should slide back in the chair.	The agreed command (e.g. 'ready, steady, slide') helps to ensure all parties make an equal effort at the same time and the effort is shared.

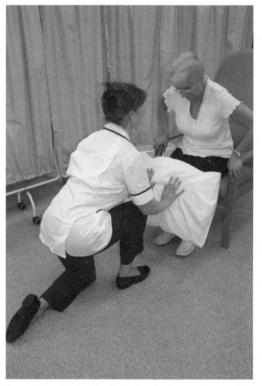

Figure 3.9   Sitting back in the chair: starting position.

Procedure Eleven   **Assisting the older person from a sitting to a standing position**

Care requirements
The older person wishes to stand from the chair but has poor thigh muscle (quadriceps) strength and needs assistance. Care should be given by an appropriately trained person.

Care objectives
To help the older person stand up from the chair. The older person will be comfortable.

Care actions	Rationale
See Symbols 1–5, Chapter 1.	
Equipment that may assist: • riser chair • handling belt may be used to give the carer a firmer hold on the older person being moved (Figure 3.10).	This may require one or two carers, based on the risk assessment of the ability of the older person.
Moving forward in the chair. The older person shuffles forward in the chair so that he/she is on the front two thirds of the seat (one third away from the back of the chair).	Natural movement requires this technique to be done in two stages. First the older person should be helped to move forwards in the chair, then helped to stand using a 'nose-over-toes' technique.
If the older person requires help to move forward in the chair, you should kneel in front of the older person and asks him/her to lean from side to side on command. Placing your hand behind the right hip, you pull the right hip forward as the older person leans towards the left.	Kneeling avoids stooping. As the older person moves from side to side they are moving the weight off the hip that you will move, reducing the effort required. A handling sling or belt will prevent twisting or over-reaching.

You then place a hand behind the left hip and pull forward as the older person leans towards the right. These alternate movements are repeated until the person to be moved is forward in the chair as described above (Figure 3.11). Alternatively, a handling sling or belt may be placed at hip height behind the person to be moved and this can be pulled from side to side (Figure 3.10).	
The carers should ensure the feet of the older person, when preparing to stand, are in an L-shaped base.	An L-shaped base increases stability.
The older person should place his/her hands on the arm of the chair to assist if possible.	
The carer(s) stand at either side of the chair with their abdomen facing the older person's shoulder.	
The carer(s) bend their knees and place their forward hand on the front of the older person's shoulder, and the other arm across the small of the older person's back with the hand on the opposite hip (Figure 3.12).	Bending the knees prevents stooping.
The designated leader checks everyone is ready and then begins to gently rock the older person to be moved giving the agreed command as the movement begins; first forward ('ready'), then back ('steady') then forward to stand ('stand').	This technique uses 'rocking' or rhythm and timing to enhance the sit to stand. The technique of rocking involves less backwards and forwards movement, preventing dizziness! The agreed command (e.g. 'ready, steady, stand') helps to ensure all parties make an equal effort at the same time and the effort is shared.
As the older person stands, gentle but firm forward and upward pressure is applied to the small of the back by the carer(s).	This enhances the natural movement used when standing of bringing the hips forward and up.

Carer(s) step forward with their front feet and bring their back feet forward by the same amount.	This ensures that a stable base is maintained throughout and carers finish in an L-shaped stable stance, not with their feet together.
Carers bring their closest hips in towards the hip of the older person and continue to hold across the small of the back to the opposite hip (Figure 3.13).	This supports the older person until they are steady on their feet.
Once the older person has stood and is stable, the hold can be relaxed and any aids given to begin walking.	

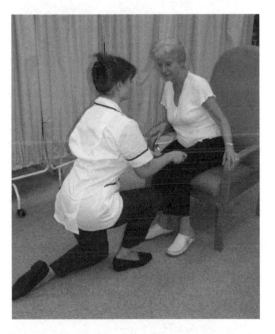

Figure 3.10 Moving forward in the chair: using a handling belt as a sling.

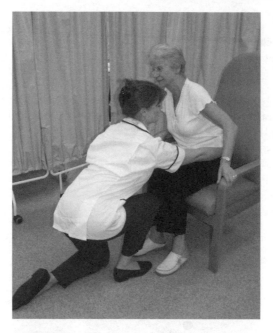

Figure 3.11 Moving forward in the chair: without a handling belt.

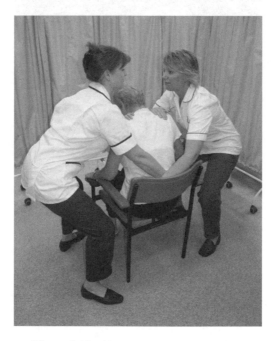

Figure 3.12 Sit to stand: starting position.

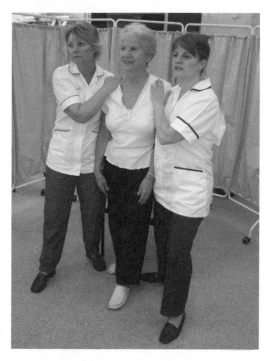

Figure 3.13   Sit to stand: finishing position – note that everyone still has an L-shaped base.

ASSISTING THE OLDER PERSON TO WALK

There are many different reasons why an older person may require assistance with walking and this is likely to be one of the most common moving and handling activities undertaken in care settings (Thomas 2005). Many things will influence an older person's ability to walk independently, including physical health, mental health and even mood. Thomas (2005) points out that while this may be a common moving and handling activity, it is also the one most associated with risk, citing the RCN's (1996) findings that 91% of reported accidents involved patients who could not walk unaided, and that half of all moving and handling accidents occurred during only three manoeuvres: the orthodox lift, the drag lift and help with walking. It is therefore clear that the carer assisting the older person should be appropriately trained in risk-reducing techniques. This section will focus on helping the older person to walk who is partly capable of performing activities of daily living independently and only requires verbal support and light physical assistance, with or without equipment. Carers may also help with walking as part of rehabilitation, but this is likely to be more risky as it often involves encouraging the older person to walk for longer or further than they previously have. In this case the assistance given and the equipment used is more specialised, requiring further knowledge.

Procedure Twelve   Assisting the older person to walk

Care requirements
The older person wishes to walk to another area/room. Care should be given by an appropriately trained person.

Care objectives
The older person will be assisted walk. The older person will be safe.

Care actions	Rationale
See Symbols 1–5, Chapter 1.	
	This technique should be used for the older person who is partly capable of performing activities of daily living independently and only requires light physical assistance and verbal support with or without equipment.
You should stand on one side of the older person, facing the direction of travel.	This prevents the carer impeding the progress of the older person.
If the older person has a walking aid, you should stand on the opposite side or, in the case of a walking frame, behind and to one side of the older person.	This allows the older person to use their walking aid appropriately.
The nearest hand to the older person may be placed on the small of the back, the hand furthest away placed on the older person's nearest shoulder or offered for support using palm-to-palm hand-hold. Do not use thumb hold (Figures 3.14, 3.15).	This provides reassurance and light support. Avoiding the thumb-hold means the hold can be released quickly if needed, preventing injury to either the carer or older person's hand. Hand-holds should be released if the older person falls while walking.

Alternatively, a palm and forearm support may be used.	This provides reassurance and should be used where the older person is taller than the carer or has painful wrists or hands.
A handling belt may be used, in which case you will hold the belt at mid-waist (Figures 3.16, 3.17).	A handling belt allows the carer to have a closer hold on the older person – but consider the need for two carers.

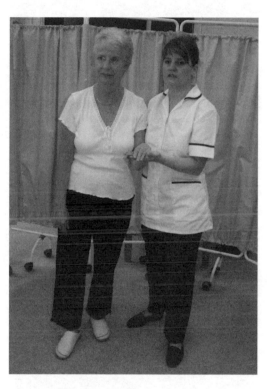

Figure 3.14   Assisted walking: palm-to-palm hold.

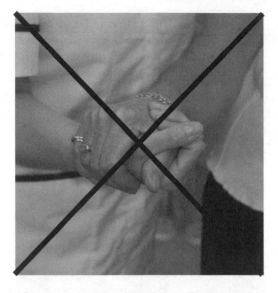

Figure 3.15   Assisted walking: thumb hold. **Do not use this method**.

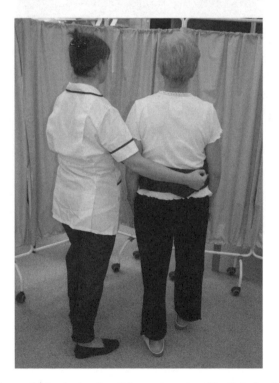

Figure 3.16   Assisted walking: using a handling belt (back).

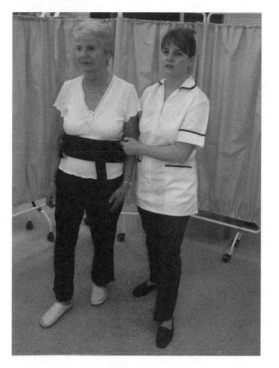

Figure 3.17 Assisted walking: using a handling belt (front).

THE FALLING PERSON

The greatest risk when assisting an older person to walk is that the older person will fall. There does not appear to be consistent advice as to what action should be taken by the carer in this situation. However, it is acknowledged by Betts and Mowbray (2005) that the risks associated with 'catching' the falling person are significant, and a high level of skill and physical fitness is required by the carer in order to manage the falling person appropriately by lowering them to the floor. It is questionable as to whether the technique of lowering a person to the floor can be adequately taught in a practical session, as the risks involved in 'practising' techniques are often considered too great. For this reason staff are usually advised not to attempt to catch, or lower the falling patient, but to provide immediate assistance once the person has fallen. This is difficult advice for the carer, but some reassurance should be taken from the information cited by Betts and Mowbray (2005) that estimates that only 5% of falls will result in a fracture.

LIFTING FROM THE FLOOR

You should never lift from the floor. If an older person has fallen to the floor you have three options:

- Give instructions to the older person to get up independently.
- Nurse the older person on the floor.
- Use a hoist to return the older person to the bed or chair.

You should *never lift* an older person – that is take the bulk of his or her body weight. If there is no alternative, and the older person needs to be lifted, then a hoist must be used.

   If you are caring for an older person in his or her own home and none of the above is possible you may need to call emergency services for assistance.

PRINCIPLES OF HOISTING

It is not possible in a book, or indeed in a training session, to explain how to safely and competently use any hoist that you may encounter. There is an ever-increasing variety of hoists available and it should be remembered that being able to use one type does not mean that you can use any type. Being hoisted can be a daunting prospect for the older person, and bad experiences of hoisting may underlie an older person's subsequent refusal to be hoisted. It is therefore important that you ensure you have received instruction about using a particular hoist before attempting to use it. There are, however, some principles that apply to all passive hoists. A passive hoist is one that lifts the entire weight of a person. A standing hoist relies on the person to be moved being able to take some weight on his/her own legs.

   Ensure you have the correct size sling for the older person. Most are marked on the sling or colour coded, with a key on the hoist itself. You can check the size by making sure the length from the top of the head (if the sling has a head support) or neck to the bottom of the spine (coccyx) is right. This can be done even when the older person is seated or lying down.

   When bringing the hoist in towards the older person, have the spreader bar, or wishbone, of the hoist at chest or abdomen level, rather than eye level which can be threatening.

   The brakes should only be applied when the hoist is not being used and is parked. This contradicts what might be thought of as safe practice but there is a good reason for this. Just like human beings, the hoist has a centre of gravity, and the centre of gravity changes and moves when a load is lifted. As the older person is lifted by the hoist, the hoist will move slightly towards him or her to adjust its centre of gravity – just like you would pull a box in towards your body to keep the load close to your centre of gravity. If the brakes were applied, instead of the hoist moving towards the older person being lifted, the older person would swing in towards the hoist. This could be a frightening experience and might cause injury, so should be avoided. Similarly, when the older person is lowered in the hoist, the hoist will move away slightly. If the brakes were to be applied there is a risk that while lowering into a chair, for example, the chair would begin to tip backwards. Again, this is frightening and potentially dangerous and should be avoided.

Most hoists have a facility to widen the legs of the hoist. This should be done whenever possible during lifting, as this gives the hoist a larger, more stable base.

Try to operate the hoist in continuous movements rather than short jerky bursts as this is more comfortable for the person being moved.

It is worth warning the older person that he or she may feel the sling slipping around him or her during the lift and that this is quite safe.

There should be two batteries for a hoist, one in the hoist and one on charge. You should know how to tell if a battery is running down (many have flashing indicator lights) and how to change the battery or use the emergency lowering system.

4 Care for the older person requiring assistance to maintain nutrition and fluid intake

Maintaining nutrition and fluid intake is essential to promote health and well-being and to aid recovery from trauma, surgery or disease. As the *National Service Framework for Older People* (DoH 2001a) points out, being overweight or underweight can have a detrimental effect on the older person's health and well-being. Being overweight can precipitate diseases such as diabetes and osteo-arthritis, and being underweight can predispose to pressure sores and delay the healing process. Poor nutritional status has been shown to delay recovery and thus lengthen hospital stay (Lennard-Jones 1992).

Factors such as social and economic circumstances or restricted mobility may affect the older person's ability to buy and cook food at home, thus contributing to malnutrition, or unhealthy eating resulting in obesity. Carers have an important role to play in the prevention of malnutrition and the promotion of healthy eating in the older person, both in hospital and in the community.

Yet there is growing evidence that malnutrition is common among older people both in the hospital and in the community, with approximately 40 per cent of older persons being under nourished on admission to hospital (Royal College of Physicians 2002; Malnutrition Advisory Group 2003). This increases with the length of hospital stay, with more than 70 per cent of older people malnourished on discharge (McWhirter and Pennington 1994) Many hospitalised older people do not receive enough calories or protein (Bond 1997). According to Age Concern (2006), six out of ten older people in hospital are at risk of being malnourished. A malnourished older person stays in hospital longer, requires more medications, is more likely to suffer from infections, complications following surgery and has a higher mortality than a well-fed older person. Age Concern believes the carer is fundamental to ending what it calls 'this scandal' by ensuring the older person receives appropriate food and help with eating. Hence this is our focus in this chapter.

As a carer you need to identify if the older person is at risk of malnutrition and help plan care to meet their needs. In addition you should ensure that the older person who is admitted to hospital well nourished does not become undernourished. If the older person is obese you may need to educate them and provide support to facilitate a change in their eating habits. On-going assessment is a key factor in ensuring that nutritional and fluid intake is adequate and appropriate in the older person. Regular weighing will help you to do this.

ASSESSING EATING AND DRINKING

Assessment of eating and drinking is part of general functional assessment. A validated nutritional screening tool such as the Malnutrition Universal Screening Tool may be used to assess and monitor the older person's nutritional status (DoH 2001b). Where appropriate, the dietitian will assess the older person's nutritional needs in relation to his or her height, weight and clinical condition. If there is any doubt about the older person's swallowing reflex, the speech and language therapist will assess swallowing and, if necessary, recommend a safe texture of food and fluids. If the older person has any special dietary requirements because of conditions such as diabetes or food allergies, or because of particular religious beliefs, this should be documented in the care plan and food and drink should comply with them. Conditions that restrict mobility such as stroke or Parkinson's Disease may affect the older person's ability and desire to eat and drink. The older person's mental state may also lead to malnutrition or obesity. Dementia, depression and reduced levels of consciousness and awareness may well affect the older person's desire and ability to eat or drink.

It is important, as a first stage, to assess how the older person manages to eat and drink. If he or she is not able to do this independently, cutlery and crockery can be adapted to help the older person maintain his or her independence. A lightweight beaker may be easier for the older person to manage than a cup and saucer or mug. A straw may make drinking easier. A plate guard may keep food from falling off the plate, and a mat under the plate may prevent the plate sliding. Cutlery can be shaped for ease of movement. The occupational therapist will be able to advise further. If the older person is likely to spill food or fluid over his or her clothes, a large absorbent serviette placed over the person's front may preserve his or her dignity and independence.

There is a varying degree of loss of taste and smell in the older person which can affect appetite (Mathey et al. 2001). The older person may like to add to taste by applying salt and pepper and spice to food. Older people tend to have a diminished taste for sweetness in food so may like strongly sweetened food. Artificial sweetness should be used to sweeten food and drink if the older person has diabetes. Oral hygiene and well-fitting dentures are also very important factors in encouraging appetite. The older person should be able to choose from a menu, if possible, what he or she likes to eat. Appetite and enjoyment of a meal will be enhanced by a comfortable, peaceful and orderly environment and an unhurried atmosphere. A variety of foods, punctual service and social companionship may also promote appetite and enjoyment. The older person should be offered the toilet or commode before his or her meal is due, so that food is not left to get cold, or the meal interrupted. The older person should be in a comfortable position, upright in a chair if possible. Food should be attractively prepared, and helpings should not be too large. Hot or cold food should be kept on plates of the correct temperature.

ASSISTING THE OLDER PERSON'S NUTRITION AND FLUID INTAKE

If an older person is unable to maintain his or her own nutritional or fluid intake you will need to assist. Assistance may take different forms according to the individual person's needs. For example, the older person may lack dexterity or movement. In this case you may need to help the older person to eat or drink.

ASSISTING AN OLDER PERSON WITH NUTRITION AND FLUID INTAKE VIA A NASOGASTRIC TUBE

If the older person cannot eat or drink orally due to inability to swallow or to reduced consciousness, he or she may require a nasogastric tube or even a permanently fitted percutanous endoscopic tube.

A nasogastric tube (NG tube) enables a nutritionally adequate diet to be delivered directly into the stomach, bypassing the oral route (Best 2005). Nasogastric tube feeding may be necessary for short-term nutritional support (up to six weeks) if the older person has a medical condition, such as loss of swallowing reflex, or reduced consciousness, that prevents nutritional needs being met by mouth. Nasogastric tube feeding may also be required if the older person needs to supplement oral intake.

A nasogastric tube is a tube that is passed through the nose and down through the nasopharynx and oesophagus into the stomach (see Diagram 5). It is a flexible tube made of rubber or plastic, and it has bidirectional potential. It can be used to remove the contents of the stomach – including air – to decompress the stomach, or to remove small solid objects and fluid, such as poison, from the stomach.

A nasogastric tube can also be used to put substances into the stomach, and so it may be used to give the older person nutrients when he or she cannot take food or drink by mouth. Enteral feeding is suitable as long as the older person has a functional gastrointestinal tract (Bowling 2004). However, the nasogastric route will not be suitable for the older person if they are at high risk of aspiration, gastric stasis, gastro-oesophageal reflux, nasal injuries or base-of-skull fractures, or for prolonged feeding.

Fine-bore nasogastric tubes should be used for nasogastric feeding. They are much smaller than the traditional larger-bored Ryle's tube, and are made of polyurethane, a much softer material which the older person will find more comfortable. The size of the tube should be either a 6 Fr or an 8 Fr. The 6 Fr can be used for standard feeds, but an 8 Fr should be used if the older person is receiving feeds that are high in fibre (Rollins 1997).

A nasogastric tube should only be inserted under direct supervision of a qualified health care practitioner. There are a number of methods, used singly or in combination, to check the position of a tube. However, a recent report shows that a

Procedure Thirteen   Assisting the older person to eat and drink

Care requirements
The older person requires assistance to eat and drink. Care should be given by an appropriately trained person.

Care objectives
The older person will be helped to eat and drink. The older person will have sufficient food and fluid intake to maintain adequate nutritional state. The older person will enjoy meals and drinks in comfort, while maintaining dignity.

Care actions	Rationale
See Symbols 1–5, Chapter 1.	Carer should wear apron for hygiene.
Help the older person to an appropriate position that is comfortable and upright. The most favourable position is at a table to participate in a communal meal. If this is not appropriate, the older person may need to have their meal in a chair or in bed.	To ensure the comfort and facilitate appetite, enjoyment and digestion of the older person.
If the older person is to have a meal by the bed or in bed, clear the bed-table and make clean area available for meal. Offer a napkin and position under chin.	To make sure that eating area is clean and hygienic.
If the older person needs assistance to eat and drink place a chair for you next to the older person.	By sitting down you will convey a more relaxed atmosphere and the older person will not feel hurried.
Collect meal and drink and cutlery on tray, and place on table or bed-table in view of the older person.	To promote the older person's dignity, so that you will not have to leave during the meal.
Ensure food and fluid is at correct temperature and appears appetising. Describe the food to the older person. Ensure food and drink is within reach, and is cut up if needed.	To tempt the appetite.

Give the older person food gently, according to requirements. Talk to the older person between mouthfuls, describing the food being given. If the older person is visually impaired, clock directions may help to locate different foods on the plate. Supervision rather than assistance may be required, in order to encourage the older person's independence.	To encourage participation, enjoyment, independence and consent.
Tailor the speed and manner in which food/drink is given according to the older person's needs, in order to create an unhurried atmosphere. Encourage without forcing food.	To encourage participation and enjoyment.
Allow the older person to chew and swallow food and breathe, before they are presented with the next mouthful. Give fluid gently as required.	To preserve the older person's comfort, enjoyment and dignity.
Remove any dribbles carefully with napkin.	To preserve the older person's dignity.
When assisting with a drink, tip the cup very gently so that the flow is controlled. A beaker with a spout or straw may aid this process, particularly if the older person is in bed.	To ensure that the flow is controlled and does not cause the older person to cough or choke.
Encouragement should be given to the older person to eat and drink, but do not press them once they have indicated that they have had sufficient. It may be necessary to offers small amounts of food and drink frequently.	This may diminish the older person's appetite.
Allow the older person to wash and dry hands and dentures if required.	To preserve the older person's comfort, cleanliness and dignity.

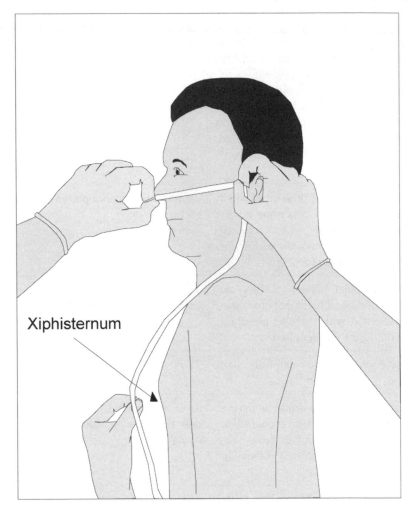

Xiphisternum

Diagram 5   Nasogastric tube position.

number of misplaced tubes have gone unnoticed (Harrison 2005). As a result, the National Patient Safety Agency (2005) has produced the following updated guidelines.

Methods that should be used to test the position of the nasogastric tube:

• Measuring the pH of aspirate using pH indicator strips/paper. PH indicator strips should have 0.5 gradients and the resulting colour change is easily distinguishable, particularly between pH 5 and pH 6.
• Radiography.

Methods that should *not* be used to test the position of the nasogastric tube:

- Auscultation of air insufflated through the nasogastric tube (whoosh test).
- Testing the acidity/alkalinity of aspirate using blue litmus paper.
- Interpreting absence of respiratory distress as an indicator of correct positioning.
- Monitoring bubbling at the end of the tube.
- Observing the appearance of feeding-tube aspirate.

The position of the tube should be checked:

- Following initial insertion.
- Before administering each feed.
- Before giving medication.
- At least once daily during continuous feeding.
- Following episodes of vomiting, retching, coughing or suctioning.

The older person who is fed via a nasogastric tube is at an increased risk of constipation and diarrhoea. Therefore it is important that you observe the frequency and consistency of the older person's faeces and liaise with a qualified health care practitioner. It may be necessary to alter the type of feed, and this may relieve the problem.

Comfort and hygiene are important considerations for the older person who has a nasogastric tube. This will include care of the facial skin on the area where the tape secures the tube to the side of the face. Nostrils will need to be cleaned daily to remove crusts and discharge. Regular oral hygiene is vital, especially if the older person is not taking anything orally.

ASSISTING AN OLDER PERSON WITH NUTRITION AND FLUID INTAKE VIA A PERCUTANOUS ENDOSCOPIC GASTROSTOMY TUBE

If nutritional support is going to be long-term then a percutanous endoscopic gastrostomy (PEG) tube is commonly used. A PEG is a feeding tube that passes through the abdominal wall directly into the stomach so that nutrition can be provided without swallowing, or in some cases to supplement oral intake (see Diagram 6). The PEG tube can be connected to a 'giving set' to provide feeds continuously, or a syringe can be used to administer bolus feeds or medication. A PEG tube is placed endoscopically by a qualified health care practitioner. PEG tubes are held in place by an internal disc and external fixation device (also called a bumper), and have a lifespan of 18–24 months. Following insertion the stoma site should not have a dressing on it. Support from a qualified health care practitioner will be needed until the stoma site is established and the older person or carer is suitably trained.

Procedure Fourteen   Nasogastric tube insertion and position checking

Care requirements
The older person is unable to swallow sufficient food and fluid and needs a nasogastric tube inserted for this purpose. Care should be given by an appropriately trained person.

Care objectives
To implement nasogastric feeding as prescribed by dietitian. The older person will be helped to maintain adequate nutrition and fluid intake. The older person will be comfortable.

Care actions	Rationale
See Symbols 1–5, Chapter 1.	This procedure should only be undertaken under direct supervision of a qualified health care practitioner.
Gather all equipment and prepare space for insertion: • nasogastric tube of appropriate size and type • lubricant • pH strips • receiver and tissues • 50 ml syringe • water (cool boiled water in the home and care home, sterile water in hospital) • gallipot • tape • clinical waste bag	To promote older person's dignity, in that you will not have to leave during the setting up of the feed. To be organised in advance in order to be more efficient.
Ensure the older person is in an appropriate position. The position of choice is for the person to be sitting upright with the head in a neutral position. If this is not possible, the older person should be lying on one side.	To maintain safety of the older person and the carer who is inserting the tube. To make insertion as easy and comfortable as possible.

Ask the older person to clear the nasal passage. Check the nostrils to determine the best one to use by asking the older person to breathe through each nostril separately to discover any blockages.	To make insertion as easy and comfortable as possible.
Open all packets of equipment, place on a clean surface, ensuring the equipment is close at hand and ready for use.	To prevent cross-infection.
Check the guide wire is not stuck within the tube by flushing with water as per manufacturer's instructions.	To aid removal of guide wire once tube has been inserted.
Estimate length of tube required, by measuring the distance from the ear lobe to nose and then nose to xiphisternum (see Diagram 5). Mark the tube if it does not already have measurements on it (as some do). If the tube has a measurement already, make a note of the length of tube to be inserted.	To ensure that tube is inserted far enough but also to ensure that excess tube is not in the stomach, as this will increase the risk of blockage.
Lubricate the tube according to manufacturer's guidelines.	To make tube insertion as easy and comfortable as possible.
Pass the tube gently into the nostril in a backwards direction along the floor of the nasopharynx. If a blockage is felt change to the other nostril (unless contra-indicated).	To aid insertion and reduce the risk of tube going into the older person's lungs.
Ask the older person to breathe through the mouth and attempt to swallow. If not contra-indicated, the older person could have sips of water via a straw. Advance the tube gently. Check to see that the tube is not going into the wrong place. Curling at the back of the throat may indicate the tube is going into the mouth. Coughing, whiteness or blueness in the face (cyanosis) may indicate that the tube is going into the bronchus. Remove the tube immediately if you see this happening, or if in any doubt.	To aid insertion and reduce the risk of tube going into the older person's lungs.

If the older person becomes distressed, stop and allow him/her time to recover before you continue to insert the tube.	To promote dignity.
When the tube has reached the measured distance, secure it temporarily by tape to the side of the face while you check its position.	To prevent the nasogastric tube from moving.
Aspirate a small amount of gastric contents (5–20 ml) from the nasogastric tube using a 50 ml syringe. Check this using pH paper that is graduated in half points. If aspirate is pH 5.5 feeding can commence. If hospital/community policy, send the older person for a chest X-ray.	To check if tube is inserted into the stomach prior to commencing feeding. Chest X-ray is the most accurate method of identifying the position of the tip of nasogastric tube. However, an X-ray will only confirm the position of nasogastric tube at the time of the X-ray. X-rays are expensive, time-consuming and impractical for the older person being cared for at home or in a community hospital. Therefore, many guidelines will allow carers to check position using pH paper.
If the contents are acidic remove the guide wire and gently secure the nasogastric tube by taping to the side of the face. Avoid tapping the tube in a manner that may cause abrasions.	To prevent the nasogastric tube becoming dislodged. Identify and record the external length markings in the older person's notes.

Procedure Fifteen   **Assisting the older person with nutrition and fluid intake via a nasogastric tube**

Care requirements
The older person is unable to swallow sufficient food and fluid and has a nasogastric tube inserted for this purpose.   Care should be given by an appropriately trained person.

Care objectives
To implement nasogastric feeding as prescribed by dietitian.   To help the older person maintain adequate nutrition and fluid intake.   To ensure the older person is comfortable.

Care actions	Rationale
See Symbols 1–5, Chapter 1.	This procedure needs further training.
Gather equipment: • nasogastric feeding pump, or reservoir bottle if a gravity method is being used • prescribed nasogastric feed • administration set • 50 ml syringe • water (cool boiled water in the home and care home and sterile in hospital) • pH strips • gloves and apron • clinical waste bag	To promote older person's dignity in that you will not have to leave during the setting up of the feed. To be organised in advance in order to be more efficient.
Ensure the older person is in an appropriate position. The position of choice is sitting in an upright position.	To maintain safety of the older person and carer. If condition permits, an upright position will aid absorption of the feed.
Check position of nasogastric tube, as in Procedure Fourteen.	To ensure nasogastric tube is in the correct position.

Flush the nasogastric tube with a minimum of 20 ml of cool boiled water or sterile water depending on local policy.	To ensure nasogastric tube is patent. As the tubes are very fine they can easily become blocked if not flushed after insertion of medication or following feeding. Sterile water or cooled boiled water should be used, as this will prevent the build-up of lime scale in the tube.
If using a bottle feed, shake container, hold bottle upright, remove the plastic cap without touching the foil seal. Do not puncture or attempt to remove the foil seal. Open the giving set and screw firmly on to the top of the bottle. Invert and hang bottle, using the integral hook.	To prevent contamination. The foil seal does not need to be removed or punctured, as the spike of the giving set will automatically break the seal.
If using a feed in a can, using a non-touch technique decant the feed into a flexi container. Open the giving set and screw firmly on to the top of the bottle. Invert and hang bottle, using the integral hook.	To prevent the risk of contamination. Non-touch technique means you do not touch openings of can or flexi container.
If using bolus feeding, attach syringe barrel without the internal piston to the nasogastric tube, using a non-touch technique. Kink the nasogastric tube to prevent the flow and fill with required fluid. Release the kink and empty gradually, raising and lowering the height of the barrel to control the speed flow. Refill and repeat until prescribed amount has been given.	To prevent the risk of contamination. Non-touch technique means you do not touch end of syringe or tube inlet.
Prime the administration set as per manufacturer's instructions allowing the feed to flow to the end.	To allow the air to be expelled.
Insert the administration set into the pump as per the manufacturer's instructions.	To ensure the pump works.

Connect administration set to nasogastric tube using a non-touch technique.	To prevent contamination.
If using a pump, set the flow rate according to the care plan, and press start. If using gravity method, adjust the roller clamp until prescribed flow rate, according to care plan, is reached.	To ensure the older person receives feed as prescribed by dietitian. Record the feed on the fluid balance chart and any other relevant documentation.
Help the older person into a comfortable position.	To maintain safety of the older person and carer.
Label administration set with date and time.	Administration sets and flexi containers should be changed every 24 hours for health and safety reasons of infection control.
When the feed is completed, or in between feeds, detach the bottle from the administration set and flush the nasogastric tube with a minimum of 30 ml water.	To prevent stasis of food and thus blockage of the nasogastric tube.

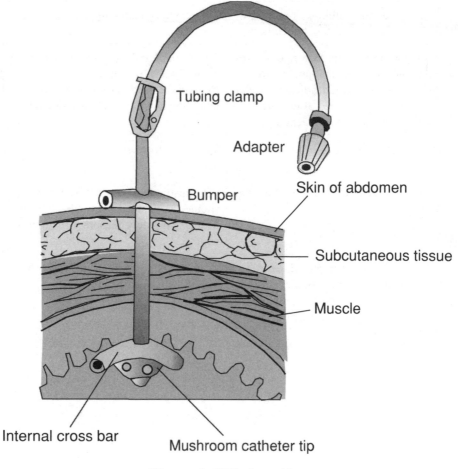

Diagram 6   PEG tube position.

POTENTIAL PROBLEMS WITH FEEDING TUBES

The most common problem with nasogastric and PEG feeding tubes is blockages. This is usually due to lack of flushing before and after administration of each dose of medication or feed. It is important to prevent tube blockage by a meticulous flushing regime. However, if a blockage does occur, try to unblock the tube by flushing with lukewarm water (Clinical Resource Efficiency Support Team (CREST) 2004; Best 2005). Do not use a syringe smaller than 50 ml as the pressure from a smaller syringe may cause the tube to burst. The water should be flushed gently into the tube. Alternatively, manufacturers may recommend a declogging agent, although pineapple juice, Coca Cola or other sugary, fizzy drinks should never be used (CREST 2004).

Procedure Sixteen   Care of percutaneous endoscopically guided gastrostomy (PEG) tube site until stoma well established (1–14 days)

Care requirements
The older person is unable to swallow food and fluid and has a percutaneous endoscopically guided gastrostomy tube (PEG) inserted for this purpose. Care should be given by an appropriately trained person.

Care objectives
The stoma site will become well established and infection free. The PEG tube should remain patent and the site should remain clean. The older person should be comfortable.

Care actions	Rationale
See Symbols 1–5, Chapter 1.	This procedure requires further training.
Gather equipment on clean trolley or tray: • sterile saline • sterile dressing pack including gallipot, swabs and gauze for dressing • sterile scissors to cut keyhole dressing • rubbish bag for debris • gloves and apron	To promote older person's dignity as you will not need to leave during the procedure. To be organised in advance in order to be more efficient.
The bumper should not be loosened or the tube rotated (see Diagram 6).	Loosening and rotation may lead the older person to develop peritonitis.
The PEG exit site should be checked daily for any erythema (redness), drainage or induration (denting).	To prevent any skin problems or dislodgement.
The stoma site should be cleaned daily with sterile saline.	To prevent any infection or irritation. An aseptic technique should be used.

If the stoma site is weeping (producing exudate), apply a dry keyhole dressing under the fixation plate. If the older person is displaying any signs of infection, such as a high temperature, a swab should be sent to microbiology for culture and sensitivity.	So that treatment can be started promptly if required. A qualified health care professional should be informed.
Ensure that the PEG tube does not become kinked or pulled.	This can cause leakage or dislodgement, which can enlarge the stoma opening or widen the stoma tract.
The stoma site should not be immersed in water until established. The older person can have a shower but not a bath. Before showering ensure the feed is disconnected and the end of the PEG is closed. Thoroughly dry the stoma site and tube following the shower.	The stoma site will not be fully healed.
If you think the PEG tube has dislodged do not use it, and contact a medical practitioner.	The tube position will need to be checked and replaced if necessary.

Procedure Seventeen   Care of percutaneous endoscopically guided gastrostomy (PEG) tube site when stoma well established

Care requirements
The older person is unable to swallow food and fluid and has a percutaneous endoscopically guided gastrostomy (PEG) tube inserted for this purpose. Care should be given by an appropriately trained person.

Care objectives
The stoma site will remain well established and infection free. The PEG tube should remain patent and the site should remain clean. The older person should be comfortable.

Care actions	Rationale
See Symbols 1–5, Chapter 1.	This procedure requires further training.
Gather equipment: • bowl of water • mild soap • disposable wipes • rubbish bag for debris • gloves and apron	To promote older person's dignity as you will not have to leave during the procedure. To be organised in advance in order to be efficient.
The bumper should be loosened and pulled back (see Diagram 11).	To facilitate the cleaning of the stoma site.
While the bumper is loosened, gently rotate the PEG 360°.	Rotation helps prevent irritation or pressure necrosis internally.
Reposition the bumper about 0.5 cm away from the abdominal wall.	If too tight it can cause skin breakdown and erythema (redness). If too loose it can cause the tube to migrate into the stomach allowing leakage of gastric content.
Clean the stoma site daily with mild soap and water. Dry with a clean towel.	To prevent infection and irritation.

Ensure that the tube is not kinked, pulled or knotted.	This can cause leakage, and dislodgement, which can enlarge the stoma opening or widen the stoma tract.
If the older person loses or gains weight the tube needs to be loosened or tightened as necessary by moving the bumper.	To maintain the older person's comfort and prevent skin breakdown.
The older person can now have a bath or a shower. They may also swim. Prior to any of these activities the tube should be closed. The site should be dried thoroughly afterwards.	The tract has now formed and the risk of accidental tube removal or dislodgement is minimal.

Procedure Eighteen   **Assisting the older person with nutrition and fluid intake via a percutaneous endoscopically guided gastrostomy (PEG) tube**

Care requirements
The older person is unable to swallow food and fluid and has a percutaneous endoscopically guided gastrostomy (PEG) tube inserted for this purpose. Care should be given by an appropriately trained person.

Care objectives
To implement PEG feeding as prescribed by dietitian. The older person will be helped to maintain adequate nutrition and fluid intake. The PEG tube should remain patent and the site should remain clean. The older person should be comfortable.

Care actions	Rationale
See Symbols 1–5, Chapter 1.	This procedure requires further training.
Gather equipment: • feeding pump, or reservoir bottle if a gravity method is being used • prescribed feed • administration set • 50 ml syringe • water (cool boiled water in the home and care home and sterile in hospital) • gloves and apron • clinical waste bag	To promote the older person's dignity as you will not need to leave during the setting up of the feed.
Ensure the older person is in an appropriate position. The position of choice is sitting in an upright position.	To maintain safety of the older person and carer. If condition permits, an upright position will aid absorption of the feed.

Flush the PEG tube with a minimum of 30 ml of cooled boiled water or sterile water according to local policy, using a 50 ml syringe.	To ensure PEG is patent. The tubes can easily become blocked if not flushed after insertion of medication or following feeding. Sterile water or cooled boiled water should be used as this will prevent the build-up of lime scale in the tube. A 20 ml or larger syringe should be used to flush the PEG tube as the pressure exerted by smaller syringes is too great.
If using a bottle feed, shake container, hold bottle upright, remove the plastic cap without touching the foil seal. Do not puncture or attempt to remove the foil seal. Open the giving set, again using a non-touch technique and screw firmly on to the top of the bottle. Invert and hang bottle, using the integral hook.	To prevent the risk of contamination. The foil seal does not need to be removed or punctured, as the spike of the giving set will automatically break the seal. Non-touch technique means you do not touch open ends of giving set or feed.
If using a feed in a can, using a non-touch technique decant the feed into a flexi container. Open the giving set, again using a non-touch technique, and screw firmly on to the top of the bottle. Invert and hang bottle, using the integral hook.	Non-touch technique is to prevent the risk of contamination.
If using bolus feeding, attach syringe barrel without the internal piston to the PEG tube, using a non-touch technique. Kink the PEG tube to prevent the flow and fill with required fluid. Release the kink and empty gradually, raising and lowering the height of the barrel to control the speed flow. Refill and repeat until prescribed amount has been given.	Non-touch technique is to prevent the risk of contamination.
If using a feeding pump, prime the administration set according to the manufacturer's instructions, allowing the feed to flow to the end.	Allow the air to be expelled to prevent air being introduced with the feed.

Insert the administration set into the pump according to the manufacturer's instructions.	To ensure the pump works.
Connect administration set to PEG tube using a non-touch technique.	Non-touch technique is to prevent the risk of contamination.
If using a pump, set the flow rate according to the care plan, and press start. If using gravity method, adjust the roller clamp until prescribed flow rate, according to care plan, is reached.	To ensure the older person receives feed as prescribed by dietitian. Record the feed on the fluid balance chart and any other relevant documentation.
Help the older person into a comfortable position.	To maintain safety of the older person and carer.
Label administration set with date and time.	Administration sets and flexi containers should be changed every 24 hours for health and safety reasons of infection control.
When the feed is completed, or in between feeds, detach the bottle from the administration set and flush the PEG tube with a minimum of 30 ml of water.	To prevent stasis of feed and thus blockage of the PEG tube.

Do not attempt to unblock a nasogastric tube by reinserting the guide wire as it may perforate the side of the tube.

Nasogastric tubes can become dislodged after coughing, vomiting or if a suctioning method has been used by the carer to remove secretions from the older person's mouth. It is important that rechecking the tube position, as explained in Procedure Fourteen, should be carried out after these events. If the older person becomes agitated and pulls the tube, or the carer feels that the exposed tube is longer than is recorded in the care plan, rechecking should take place. If the tube needs to be replaced, a suitably qualified health care practitioner should remove the tube completely, reinsert the guidewire and replace it.

PEG tubes can sometimes leak because the tube or Y adapter at the end of the PEG tube is cracked. If it is the Y adaptor that is cracked, you can replace it; if it is the tube that is cracked, fit another Y adapter beyond the crack. Because of this potential hazard it is essential that the carer always has easy access to an appropriate adapter of the correct size. The adapter needs to be carefully fitted by a trained carer, as a good seal is essential to maintain the inflation of the internal retention bumper.

If a PEG tube becomes dislodged before the tract has formed, it can result in peritonitis. This situation should be treated as an emergency (CREST 2004; Holmes 1999). If a PEG tube is dislodged after the tract has formed, the stoma will start to close within two to three hours. Therefore a suitably qualified care practitioner should refit a replacement tube as soon as possible.

5 Care for the older person requiring assistance with toilet needs

Respecting the older person's dignity and privacy is important when assisting with toilet needs (DoH 2001a). Safety is also an important consideration. If an older person is frail and unwell it is important that you help maintain independence wherever possible, while ensuring that you give appropriate assistance where required. The older person should, if possible, be left alone during elimination, with the door shut and a sign showing 'engaged'. In hospital or care home, if the older person cannot use the toilet but needs to use a bedpan or urinal in bed, a commode by the bed, or a catheter bag requires emptying, the screen needs to be drawn, or doors shut on side rooms. Similarly, if the older person is at home, the door to the room should be kept closed. Always consider if the older person can go to the toilet. It may be preferable to assist the older person with a wheelchair to visit the toilet rather than to use a commode by the bed. Follow the older person's preferences wherever you can.

As far as possible, noises of elimination should be hidden, and odours and smells reduced by air fresheners. Hygiene and the prevention of cross-infection are crucial, and the older person should be offered hand-washing facilities after performing toilet functions. Carers too should ensure they wash their hands thoroughly. Commodes, bedpans and urinals should be cleaned in line with local policy in hospital units or in the home, with detergent and hot water after each use, ensuring the underside and crevices are clean, to prevent cross-infection.

ASSISTING THE MAINTENANCE OF CONTINENCE

Many older people experience problems maintaining bladder and bowel control although these problems are not inevitable with old age. Neurological degeneration due to ageing leads to a loss of bladder muscle tone (Coni & Webster 1998), which can lead to symptoms of urgency and frequency or an inability to empty the bladder completely. Problems with mobility and toilet accessibility may combine, resulting in incontinence when an older person cannot reach the toilet in time. Functional incontinence such as this can be exacerbated in hospital or care homes if assistance does not come promptly. Medications that aid sleeping, such as sedatives and hypnotics, can mean that the older person does not wake to signals that his or her bladder needs to be emptied. This can therefore lead to night-time incontinence (Caird & Grimley Evans 1995).

Older women are prone to urinary tract infection, hormonal changes and vaginal atrophy that can aggravate continence problems. Therefore care needs to be taken with vaginal hygiene to prevent bacteria being spread from the bowel to the urethral area. Urinary tract infections can also occur where the bladder does not empty completely. This occurs in older people who have neurological problems such as stroke or multiple sclerosis but can also occur in older men due to prostate enlargement. Infection may be present without any symptoms, but symptoms can include increased body temperature, incontinence, drowsiness or mental disorientation and confusion. Prostate enlargement can lead to obstruction of the bladder neck, stasis of urine and retention, causing overflow incontinence.

Some incontinence problems can be treated easily. This can include ensuring the older person is not constipated, treating any urinary tract infections, teaching pelvic floor exercises, bladder retraining and medication. However, for some older people an appropriate management strategy needs to be found, aided by pad and pants, accessible toilet facilities and regular offers of assistance. Penile sheaths are a good alternative for men. Although an in-dwelling catheter may be required for some older people, in-dwelling catheters require careful consideration of the older person's ability to care for the drainage system independently or the availability of carers and should be discussed in full with the older person and their carers, as should all treatment options.

PREVENTING CONSTIPATION

Constipation becomes more common in older people because of the loss of muscle tone in the bowel. The older person often experiences difficulty passing stools, which can lead to the bowels being opened with less frequency. Constipation has many causes. In the older person causes include: poor appetite; inability to afford, shop for, or cook food; poor fluid intake; lack of exercise. Dementia and depression can affect appetite and motivation to shop and cook. Many older people take medications that can lead to constipation, and regular reviews of medication should be undertaken to avoid taking too many inappropriate medicines. The Bristol Stool Form Scale (Figure 5.1) (O'Donnell, Virjee & Heaton 1990; Norgine Pharmaceuticals Limited, 2000) is a useful tool for assessing the older person's normal bowel habits, and any changes.

Neglecting the feeling to open one's bowels can be caused by a lack of available help to get to the toilet, but also when passing stools becomes painful due to piles or fissures. If an older person does become constipated, a review of these issues is important before resorting to the use of laxatives. Oral laxatives provide a short-term solution to an acute constipation problem, but should be avoided in the long term. Rectal enemas and suppositories should only be prescribed when all else has failed and the older person will usually require assistance to administer these. A comprehensive assessment of the bowel function should be undertaken before any laxatives are prescribed, as inappropriate use can aggravate the problem and lead to faecal incontinence. The administration of enemas and suppositories should only be performed by a trained person and should be overseen by the registered nurse.

THE BRISTOL STOOL FORM SCALE

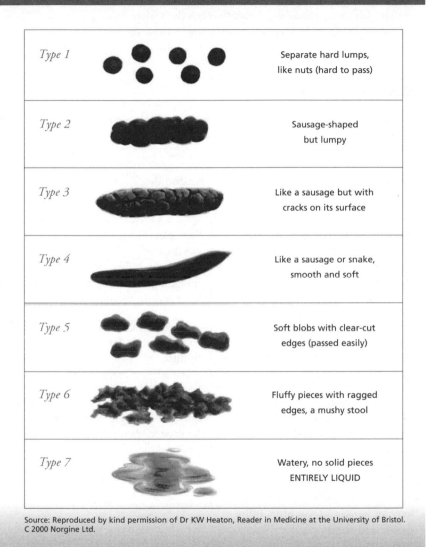

Type 1	Separate hard lumps, like nuts (hard to pass)
Type 2	Sausage-shaped but lumpy
Type 3	Like a sausage but with cracks on its surface
Type 4	Like a sausage or snake, smooth and soft
Type 5	Soft blobs with clear-cut edges (passed easily)
Type 6	Fluffy pieces with ragged edges, a mushy stool
Type 7	Watery, no solid pieces ENTIRELY LIQUID

Source: Reproduced by kind permission of Dr KW Heaton, Reader in Medicine at the University of Bristol. C 2000 Norgine Ltd.

Figure 5.1

Procedure Nineteen   Assisting the older person to use toilet, commode or bedpan

Care requirements
The older person requires assistance to reach the toilet. Care should be given by an appropriately trained person.

Care objectives
The older person will be helped to reach the toilet or use a commode or bedpan.

Care actions	Rationale
See Symbols 1–5, Chapter 1.	
According to his/her level of mobility, walk older person – or if required help older person into wheelchair and wheel them – to toilet. Ensure that you adhere to moving and handling policies at all times.	To maintain the older person's privacy and dignity. To ensure safety of the older person, yourself and any other carer(s) involved by preventing injury.
If there is restricted mobility, screen older person and make sure privacy is protected throughout procedure.	To maintain older person's privacy and dignity.
If using commode/bedpan by or in bed, collect all equipment by bedside: • either commode and lid or bedpan and cover • toilet paper • bowl of water, soap and wipes • moving and handling aids according to older person's level of mobility • gloves and apron	To promote older person's dignity, in that you will not have to leave during the procedure.
If transferring older person to commode, transfer according to moving and handling assessment. If needed, synchronise move using second or third carer and possibly hoist.	To ensure safety and prevent injury of older person, yourself and any other carer(s) assisting.

To insert a bedpan, ask the older person to bridge his/her back while lying flat, by lifting their hips up off the bed with their knees bent and feet, forearms and palms flat on the bed. They can then push down on their forearms and feet to lift their bottom, while the carer inserts the bedpan. If the older person is unable to bridge his/her back unaided, at least two carers will be needed. In this case identify who will lead the move and adjust bed to appropriate height – between hip and waist for rolling. Then carry out the manoeuvres below.	To promote independence of the older person.
• Position the older person's arms on the chest. The nearside arm should be bent at the elbow and upper forearm should be pointing towards head of bed and parallel to older person's shoulders. Furthest leg is bent at knee or crossed over nearside leg. • Turn older person's head in direction of movement. • To roll the older person, position your feet one foot in front of the other, with knees slightly bent. • On command 'ready, steady, roll', you straighten knees to upright position or use weight-transfer technique by rocking from front leg on to back leg. Roll older person to side and insert pan. • To put back, reverse the procedure.	To promote safety and prevent injury to older person, yourself and any other carer(s) assisting.
If transferring to toilet or commode and older person is able to bear weight, one or two carers to stand at side of older person, facing forward. Once he or she is standing, a walking frame or grab rail may be used to support balance. If the older person is not able to bear weight a hoist or transfer board should be used.	To promote safety and prevent injury to older person, yourself and any other carer(s) assisting.

Make sure the older person is comfortable and safe while on toilet, commode or bedpan. Ensure brakes are applied on commode wheels. Assess any risks (e.g. falling). Ask older person if she/he would like to be left alone and agree a time limit. If so, ensure call bell to summon assistance is within reach. When older person has finished, offer toilet paper and help to use it if necessary.	Re-evaluate risk throughout the procedure. To preserve older person's comfort, dignity and safety.
If using toilet or commode, and the older person is able, help them to move forward on the toilet seat, then back against the cistern or back rest.	This action opens the angle of the hips, giving more space for the older person wishing to clean the frontal area. For this reason it is easier if the toilet seat has a dipped access area at the front of the seat. From the forward seated position, the older person can be helped to lean forward, giving a larger space behind, to help you to clean the older person's anal region. This approach can usually be done with one carer and helps the older person retain privacy and dignity.
Offer older person water, soap and wipes to wash and dry hands.	To maintain older person's comfort and dignity and prevent cross-infection.
Assist older person back to wheelchair, chair or bed, adhering to moving and handling regulations.	To prevent harm or injury to older person, yourself and any other carers assisting.

Observe faecal/urinary colour, consistency, amount and foreign matter.	To monitor older person's condition and evaluate any change in bowel motion or urine.
	Normal faeces should be brown, soft and formed and have an odour but should not be offensive. Note the amount of faeces passed, the consistency and colour, how often the bowels are opened, and any pain or discomfort experienced when passing the stool.
	Normal urine is straw-coloured and should be free of particles and debris. Dark yellow urine indicates that it is more concentrated than normal. A 'fishy' smell may indicate a urine infection.

**Procedure Twenty   Assisting the older person requiring bowel care:
administration of suppositories**

Care requirements
The older person needs assistance to open his/her bowels. Care should be given by an appropriately trained person.

Care objectives
The older person will have his/her bowels open. The older person will feel comfortable.

Care actions	Rationale
See Symbols 1–5, Chapter 1.	This procedure needs further training.
Collect equipment required for procedure: • clean tray • disposable incontinence pad • topical swabs or tissues • lubricating jelly • commode preferably (bedpan if bedbound) to be placed nearby • toilet paper • suppository (suppositories) as prescribed by a doctor or nurse • gloves and apron • clinical waste bag	Promote the older person's dignity, in that you will not have to leave during the procedure. To be organised in advance in order to be efficient. The incontinence pad may be needed in case of premature ejaculation of suppositories, or rapid bowel movement following administration. A commode is preferable to a bedpan because it requires less straining during evacuation owing to gravity.
Screen older person and make sure privacy is protected throughout procedure. Adjust bed to comfortable working height if possible.	To protect the older person's dignity and avoid unnecessary embarrassment. To minimise strain on yourself.
Help older person to lie in correct position, adhering to moving and handling regulations. Assistance from another carer may be required. Position of choice is for the older person to be on their left side with knees flexed, one above the other, with the buttocks near the edge of the bed.	Allows ease of passage of the suppository into the rectum. Flexing the knees will reduce discomfort as the suppository passes through the anal sphincter.

Place absorbent pad under older person.	To avoid embarrassment to older person of soiled linen.
If constipation is established, lubricate with lubricating gel either blunt or pointed end of suppository, according to manufacturer's guidelines.	Lubricating reduces friction and so eases insertion of the suppository and avoids damage to anal mucosa. There is professional disagreement about the correct method for inserting suppositories (whether blunt or pointed end first). Manufacturer's information should be followed at all times to adhere to legal terms of the product licence.
Part the buttocks with one hand and gently insert the suppository with your index finger of the other hand. The suppository should be inserted approx 4 cm. Repeat if second suppository is prescribed.	To promote the older person's comfort. The anal canal is 2–4 cm long. Inserting the suppository beyond this makes sure that it will be retained and absorbed.
Once suppository has been inserted, clean any excess lubricating jelly from the older person's perineal area.	To make sure older person is comfortable and to avoid anal excoriation which may lead to infection.
Cover older person with sheet/blanket.	To maintain comfort and dignity.
Ask the older person to retain suppository (suppositories) for 20 minutes, or until no longer able to do so. They should remain lying down.	This will allow suppository to melt and release the active ingredients.
Adjust height of bed. Provide a call bell at hand. Make sure assistance is available if older person needs help to get to commode/toilet.	To ensure height of bed facilitates the older person's safety both in bed and when he/she transfers out of bed. To make sure older person is comfortable and to minimise anxiety.
When required, help older person on to commode/bedpan, as described in Procedure Nineteen.	To maintain older person's privacy, dignity and comfort.
Document and report result.	To plan care.

Procedure Twenty-one   Assisting the older person requiring bowel care: administration of an evacuant enema

Care requirements
The older person needs assistance to open his/her bowels. Care should be given by an appropriately trained person.

Care objectives
The older person will have his/her bowels open. The older person will feel comfortable.

Care actions	Rationale
See Symbols 1–5, Chapter 1.	This procedure needs further training.
Collect equipment: • clean tray • apron and gloves • disposable incontinence pad • topical swabs or tissues • lubricating jelly • commode preferably (bedpan if bed-bound) to be placed nearby • toilet paper • enema as prescribed by a doctor or a nurse	Promote older person's dignity, in that you will not have to leave during the procedure. To be organised in advance in order to be efficient. The incontinence pad may be needed in case of rapid bowel movement following administration of enema. A commode is preferable to a bedpan because it requires less straining during evacuation owing to gravity.
Screen older person and make sure privacy is protected throughout procedure. Adjust bed to comfortable working height if possible.	To protect the older person's dignity and avoid unnecessary embarrassment. To minimise strain on yourself.
Help older person to lie in correct position, adhering to moving and handling regulations. Assistance from another carer may be required. Position of choice is for the older person to be on their left side with knees flexed, one above the other, with the buttocks near the edge of the bed. Place absorbent pad under older person.	Allows ease of passage of the enema into the rectum. Flexing the knees will reduce discomfort as the enema passes through the anal sphincter. To avoid embarrassment to older person of soiled linen.

Warm the enema to body temperature by immersing in a jug of hot water.	Heat is an effective stimulant of the nerves in the intestinal mucosa. An enema of body temperature will not damage the intestinal mucosa. The temperature of the environment, the rate of fluid administration, and length of tubing all affect temperature of fluid in rectum.
If constipation is established, expel any air from enema container and lubricate enema nozzle with lubricating gel, separate the older person's buttocks and touch the anal sphincter to stimulate contraction. As sphincter relaxes tell older person to breathe deeply through mouth as you gently insert tube 5 cm.	Expel air in order to prevent the introduction of air into the colon which can cause distension and discomfort. Lubricating reduces friction and so eases insertion of the nozzle and avoids damage to anal mucosa. Allowing the sphincter to relax eases the passage of the tube.
If pain occurs or resistance is felt at any time during the procedure, consider whether the older person is unable to relax or has spasm: a) Encourage older person to take deep breaths, 'bear down' as if defecating. b) Allow a little solution to flow, then insert tube 5 cm further. c) If in doubt, stop and seek medical advice.	a) The older person may be apprehensive and tense and unable to relax anal sphincter. b) There may be a faecal blockage. c) A tumour may be causing a blockage.
Introduce the fluid slowly by rolling the pack from the bottom to the top to prevent back flow, until the solution is finished.	The faster the rate of flow of the fluid, the greater the pressure on the rectal walls. Distension and irritation of the bowel wall will produce strong peristalsis which is sufficient to empty the lower bowel.
Slowly withdraw the nozzle, and clean any excess lubricating jelly from the older person's perineal area.	To avoid reflex emptying of rectum. To make sure older person is comfortable and to avoid anal excoriation which may lead to infection.

Ask the older person to retain enema for 30 minutes, or until no longer able to do so. The older person should remain lying down.	This will enhance the evacuant effect.
Adjust bed height. Provide a call bell at hand. Make sure help is available if older person needs assistance to get to commode/toilet.	To ensure height of bed facilitates older person's safety both in bed and when he/she transfers out of bed. To make sure the older person is comfortable and to minimise anxiety. The procedure may make an older person feel weak or faint.
When required, help older person on to commode/bedpan as described in Procedure Nineteen.	To maintain the older person's privacy, dignity and comfort.
Document and report result.	To plan care.

Procedure Twenty-two   Obtaining a specimen of faeces for observation, assessment and analysis

Care requirements
A specimen of the older person's faeces is required for observation, assessment and analysis. Care should be given by an appropriately trained person.

Care objectives
A specimen of the older person's faeces will be collected, observed, assessed and analysed. The older person will understand the reason for the procedure. The older person will be comfortable throughout the procedure.

Care actions	Rationale
See Symbols 1–5, Chapter 1.	
Collect equipment and place in either the bathroom or by the older person's bedside: • clinically clean bedpan/slipper pan. You will also need the following equipment. However, if you are in a hospital environment you would leave this in the sluice: • clinically clean container with spatula, if not already attached in specimen container • sterile specimen container labelled with older person's details, completed pathology request form, specimen bag • bedpan/slipper pan and cover • gloves and apron • clinical waste bag	To maintain older person's dignity, in that you do not have to leave during the procedure. To be organised in advance in order to be efficient.

According to the older person's level of mobility, help the older person to the toilet. If restricted mobility, use most appropriate toilet aid.	To make sure older person's privacy, dignity and comfort are maintained. To ensure safety and prevent harm to the older person, yourself and any other carers involved.
Collect faeces in bedpan/slipper pan. Cover when removed from older person.	So that you can assess and monitor bowel habits and take a sample for analysis. To ensure older person's dignity. Potential biohazard if spilled.
Offer older person hand wash. As required, help older person back to chair/bed and into a comfortable position.	To maintain older person's comfort and dignity.
Return to the faeces and either take to the sluice or bathroom. Observe the faeces so that you can record normal pattern of defecation. Use Bristol Stool Form Scale to assess appearance and frequency of faeces (Figure 5.1). Colour may indicate bleeding in gastrointestinal tract: upper tract – black and tarry with odour (malaena); lower tract – maroon; local in anus – bright red; obstructed bile – putty coloured. Iron therapy gives odourless slate-grey/black stool.	To adhere to good recording and documentation legislation and to monitor any change in the older person's bowel habits. If any abnormalities found, ensure you report to appropriate health care professional so that treatment can begin if appropriate. These are possible indications only.
Use spatula to remove a small usable amount of the faeces (to fill about a third of the container). Put specimen into sterile container.	To have a usable amount of specimen for investigation.
Ensure the older person's name, address or ward, and date and time are recorded on pathology request form. Place sealed container in specimen bag with form. If specimen bag is transparent ensure person's details are not visible through the bag. Send as soon as possible to pathology.	To ensure correct information is given to the laboratory. To preserve confidentiality. If kept at room temperature organisms multiply and lead to misinterpretation of results.

Procedure Twenty-three   Obtaining a specimen of urine for observation, assessment and analysis

Care requirements
A specimen of the older person's urine is required for observation, assessment and analysis. Care should be given by an appropriately trained person.

Care objectives
A specimen of the older person's urine will be collected, observed, assessed and analysed. The older person will understand the reason for the procedure. The older person will be comfortable throughout the procedure.

Care actions	Rationale
See Symbols 1–5, Chapter 1.	
Collect equipment and place in either the bathroom or by the older person's bedside: • clinically clean bedpan or bottle, if person is unable to use toilet • soap and water or 0.9% saline and disposable/clean cloth • sterile specimen container labelled with older person's details • completed pathology request form • specimen bag • gloves and apron • clinical waste bag	To maintain older person's dignity, in that you do not have to leave during the procedure. To be organised in advance in order to be efficient.
According to the older person's level of mobility, help her/him to the toilet. If restricted mobility, use most appropriate toilet aid.	To make sure the older person's privacy, dignity and comfort are maintained at all times. To ensure safety and prevent harm to the older person, yourself and any other carers involved.

To obtain mid-stream specimen of urine, collect as soon as possible after older person has woken. Ask her/him to clean around urethral meatus, or help to clean, with soap and water or 0.9% saline. (In men, retract prepuce.) Use cloth once only, and clean from front to back. Pat dry with a clean towel. Ask older person to start urinating into bottle, bedpan or toilet, but to direct middle part of flow into sterile container, and finish urinating in bottle, bedpan or toilet. If older person is unable to do this, specimen will need to be taken from bedpan/urinal.	Urine passed overnight will be undiluted. To ensure older person's dignity. Antiseptic should not be used because of contamination. To flush residue before collecting specimen. Potential biohazard if spilled.
Offer older person hand wash. As required, help older person back to chair/bed and into a comfortable position.	To prevent harm or injury to the older person, yourself and any other carers assisting. To maintain older person's comfort and dignity.
Return to the urine and either take to the sluice or bathroom. If older person was unable to urinate into sterile container pour a small usable amount into sterile container (20 ml).	To have a usable amount of specimen for investigation.
Pour remainder of urine into clear container. Assess for macroscopic appearance: • cloudy – settlement of sediment and infection • milky – infection, chluria, spermatozoa, urate crystals, insoluble phosphates • blue/green – pseudomonas, bilirubin • pink/red – blood, drugs, beetroot • orange – drugs • yellow and brown – bilirubin • brown/black – blood Assess urine for odour – if left to stand smells of ammonia; if infected smells fishy; if it contains ketones smells sweet. Assess for volume: average output 1500 ml per 24 hours.	To adhere to good recording and documentation legislation and to monitor change. If any abnormalities found, ensure you report to appropriate health care professional so that treatment can begin if appropriate. These are possible indications only.

Test with urinalysis stick by dipping stick into a fresh, well mixed sample of urine; withdraw stick and wipe along rim of container to remove excess urine; compare with colour chart on side of container for specified time: • presence of glucose – diabetes, Cushing's syndrome, acute pancreatitis • presence of ketones – starvation, diabetes • presence of protein – renal disease, urinary tract infection, congestive heart failure • presence of blood – trauma, infection, renal stones, drugs • presence of bilirubin – hepatic or biliary disease, stale urine • raised urobilinogen – liver disease, haemolytic anaemia • presence of nitrites – urinary tract infection • presence of leucocytes – urinary tract infection • pH greater than 7 (acidic) may indicate infection and fever	To monitor change. If any abnormalities found ensure you report to appropriate health care professional so that treatment can begin if appropriate. These are possible indications only.
Ensure the older person's name, address or ward, and date and time are recorded on pathology request form. Place sealed container in specimen bag with form. If specimen bag is transparent ensure person's details are not visible through the bag. Send as soon as possible to pathology.	To ensure correct information is given to the laboratory. To preserve confidentiality. If kept at room temperature organisms multiply, which leads to misinterpretation of results.

ASSISTING THE OLDER PERSON WITH AN IN-DWELLING CATHETER

The older person may have an in-dwelling urinary catheter. This is a catheter that is inserted into the bladder in order to evacuate urine (Dougherty & Lister 2004; Baillie 2005). The urinary catheter is a long, hollow drainage tube made of a synthetic substance such as silicone. It has a balloon that, when in place, is inflated with a small amount of sterile water to hold it there. An in-dwelling catheter can be left *in situ* long term or for a period of time while the older person is recovering from an illness. The older person may have an in-dwelling catheter inserted for a number of reasons, for example to relieve urinary retention or to relieve incontinence when no other means is practicable. There is a range of catheters on the market, and careful assessment of the older person will need to be carried out by a qualified health care practitioner in order to ensure that the most appropriate material, size and balloon capacity is selected to ensure that the catheter is as effective as possible and complications are minimised (Dougherty & Lister 2004; Baillie 2005).

In-dwelling catheters are used in conjunction with a drainage bag, which allows for emptying but at the same time ensures a closed system. The older person may prefer the catheter to drain into a leg bag, which attaches to the leg or thigh with velcro straps, and is therefore hidden by clothing. This protects the older person's privacy and dignity. It will also aid the older person's mobilisation. The other form of drainage bag is a bed bag, which is larger than the leg bag, holds more urine and has a longer tube. The bed bag can be fixed to a holder that attaches to the bed or a chair or is placed on the floor. This has the advantage of holding more urine, but is more visible than the leg bag and more restrictive of movement, because it needs to be carried if the older person walks. It may, however, be more comfortable for the older person overnight, enabling movement in bed, and because it holds a larger quantity of urine than the leg bag.

The main complication with in-dwelling urinary catheterisation is infection (Wilde 1997; Dougherty & Lister 2004; Baillie 2005). A study carried out in 1957 (Macauley 1997) found that prior to the closed system nearly 100 per cent of patients developed a urinary tract infection. However, the closed system still has many entry points for bacteria. While the older person has an in-dwelling catheter in place the bladder's normal closing mechanism is obstructed by the catheter and thus the natural flushing mechanism when passing urine is lost (Baillie 2005). As the catheter is close to the bowel there is potential for infection as bacteria can be mechanically transferred across the skin surfaces. It is therefore extremely important that either the older person, if able, or you as the carer, maintains high levels of standard precautions when carrying out catheter care (DoH 2005c).

Another complication associated with in-dwelling catheters is encrustation of the catheter, which can eventually lead to blockage. If this happens, advice and assistance will need to be obtained from an appropriately trained health care professional.

Catheter care includes cleaning the urethral meatus (the point where the catheter enters the body), emptying the catheter bag, changing the catheter bag and taking a catheter specimen of urine (CSU). The older person can be taught to do this himself or herself, if able. If this is not possible or desirable, as the carer you will need to assist. The urethral meatus of the older person should be washed with water twice daily and following bowel actions in order to reduce the risk of infection. Catheter bags should be emptied when the catheter bag is three quarters full. Emptying more frequently will increase the risk of infection as you are opening the closed system unnecessarily. Allowing the catheter bag to become more than three quarters full will increase the risk of infection if the urine back-tracks up the catheter and passes into the bladder again. A catheter drainage bag should be selected for length, style and type according to the older person's needs. At present there does not appear to be specific research that recommends how often catheter bags should be changed. However, disconnection of the catheter from the drainage bag significantly increases the risk of introducing bacteria into the system and should therefore be done as infrequently as possible (Wilson 1997). The DoH (1999) recommends that catheter bags be changed every five to seven days, or if damaged or blocked with deposits. When assisting the older person to change the catheter bag it is important that you reduce the risk of infection by maintaining high standards of hygiene.

It is recommended that anyone with an in-dwelling catheter has an adequate fluid intake (providing his or her condition allows for this). This will dilute the urine, leaving it with fewer nutrients and discouraging the growth of bacteria (Wilson 1997; Baillie 2005). The recommended amount of fluid intake is 2–2.5 litres per 24 hours.

General care of the older person with an in-dwelling catheter also includes observing him or her for signs of infection, and reporting any pyrexia, discomfort, drowsiness or changes in mental state to the health care professional. These signs and symptoms could indicate an infection. If this happens, a catheter specimen of urine (CSU) should be obtained. This should be analysed with a urinalysis strip and, if abnormality or infection is indicated, sent to the microbiology laboratory for further analysis. At the laboratory the specimen will be checked to see what organisms are present and how they can be treated (culture and sensitivity). You should also observe and record how much urine is passed (urine output), that urine is draining, that the catheter is not blocked or leaking, that the catheter is in place, and that there is no bleeding from the catheter.

As always, all details of care should be documented. Before helping the older person to care for his or her catheter it is important that you check in the care plan the date that the catheter was inserted, the size and type of catheter, the patency and amount and colour of urine output, and when the catheter drainage bag was last changed. Catheter bags should be positioned in such a way as to allow drainage by gravity and so avoid reflux of urine back up the tube. The bag should not touch the floor or any other sources of contamination. Catheters should be changed according to type and manufacturer's recommendations: short term (1–14 days); short to medium term (2–6 weeks); medium to long term (6 weeks–3 months). These points are important as they will help maintain the older person's comfort and dignity and help prevent urinary tract infections.

Procedure Twenty-four   Assisting the older person with catheter care

Care requirements
The older person has an in-dwelling catheter. Care should be given by an appropriately trained person.

Care objectives
The risk of urinary tract infection will be minimised. The catheter will remain patent. The older person will feel comfortable.

Care actions	Rationale
See Symbols 1–5, Chapter 1.	
Collect the equipment required: • wash-bowl with warm water • mild soap if required • disposable cloths • towel • clinical waste bag to dispose of wipes as per local policy • gloves and apron	To maintain older person's dignity so that you do not have to leave during the procedure. To be organised in advance in order to be efficient.
Help the older person into an appropriate position. If the older person is in bed the best position, if possible, is supine, with knees and hips flexed and slightly apart. Ensure that you adhere to moving and handling regulations.	To prevent harm or injury to older person, yourself and any other carers assisting. To maintain older person's comfort and dignity.
For the female older person: With a disposable cloth, warm water and soap, wash the peri-anal area by wiping from front to back. Repeat, if required, ensuring you use a new disposable cloth each time.	Cleaning from front to back will reduce the risk of transfer of micro-organisms from the bowel to the catheter entry. Cleaning with soap and water is as effective as any other method in reducing infection and removing secretions and encrustations. Each cloth should be used only once, to prevent the spread of micro-organisms.

With a new disposable cloth and warm water rinse the older female's peri-anal area by wiping from front to back to remove the soap.	If soap is not rinsed off it can cause irritation and sore skin.
For the male older person: Retract the foreskin and wash the penis away from the meatal junction with a disposable cloth, warm water and soap.	Cleaning away from the meatal junction will reduce the risk of transfer of micro-organisms. Cleaning with soap and water is as effective as any other method in reducing infection and removing secretions and encrustations. Each cloth should be used only once to prevent the spread of micro-organisms.
With a new disposable cloth and warm water rinse the penis by wiping away from the meatal junction to remove the soap.	Soap, if not rinsed off, can cause irritation and sore skin.
For the female older person, with a clean cloth, soap and water clean the shaft of the catheter by gently wiping in one direction away from the vulva and meatal junction. For the male older person, with a clean cloth, soap and water clean the shaft of the catheter by gently wiping in one direction away from the meatal junction.	Cleaning away from the meatal junction will reduce the risk of transfer of micro-organisms.
With a new disposable cloth rinse the catheter shafts as above. For the male older person ensure that you replace the foreskin.	Soap if not rinsed off, can cause irritation and sore skin.
Dry the older person by patting with a clean towel.	To prevent the risk of micro-organisms, as they will grow on warm moist skin. Skin will become sore if not dried.

Procedure Twenty-five   Assisting the older person to empty a catheter bag

Care requirements
The older person has an in-dwelling catheter. Care should be given by an appropriately trained person.

Care objectives
The risk of urinary tract infection will be minimised. The catheter will remain patent. The older person will feel comfortable.

Care actions	Rationale
See Symbols 1–5, Chapter 1.	
Collect the equipment required: • clean disposable urinal or jug and cover • clean catheter bag if required • either a swab saturated with isopropyl alcohol 70%, or isopropyl alcohol 70% spray • gloves and apron • clinical waste bag	To maintain the older person's dignity, in that you will not have to leave during the procedure. To be organised in advance in order to be efficient. If non-disposable jug is used to collect urine it should be used only for this purpose, to prevent cross-infection.
Screen bed. If older person is in bed, adjust bed to comfortable working height.	To protect older person's dignity and privacy. To minimise strain on individuals.
Spray outlet tap with 70% isopropyl alcohol spray or wipe outlet tap with swab soaked in 70% isopropyl alcohol; allow to dry for 30 seconds before opening.	To reduce the risk of bacteria entering the closed system. This is a non-touch technique. The highest risk of cross-infection occurs when a catheter drainage bag is emptied or changed.
Drain catheter bag into a clean disposable urinal or jug, ensuring that the tap does not touch the container, your hands or the floor and cover.	To reduce the risk of bacteria entering the closed system. To prevent cross-infection.

Close the tap and either spray it with 70% isopropyl alcohol spray or wipe it with a new swab soaked in 70% isopropyl alcohol.	To reduce the risk of bacteria entering the closed system.
Ensure the drainage bag is kept below the level of the bladder and does not touch the floor. If using a leg bag ensure the bag is strapped securely to the older person's leg without causing tension or abrasion.	To prevent contamination and cross-infection. To promote comfort and ensure drainage.
Take covered jug or bottle to sluice or toilet. Measure urine if required. Observe urine for consistency, colour, odour and debris.	To monitor output and consistency of urine. To monitor for signs of infection.

Procedure Twenty-six   Obtaining a catheter specimen of urine for observation, assessment and analysis

Care requirements
A specimen of the older person's urine is required for observation, assessment and analysis. Care should be given by an appropriately trained person.

Care objectives
A specimen of the older person's urine will be collected, observed, assessed and analysed. The older person will understand the reason for the procedure. The older person will be comfortable throughout the procedure.

Care actions	Rationale
See Symbols 1–5, Chapter 1.	
Collect equipment and place in either the bathroom or by the older person's bedside: • clean tray • either a swab saturated with 70% isopropyl alcohol or 70% isopropyl alcohol spray • gate clip • sterile syringe (20 ml) and 25 g needle (orange) if required • sterile specimen container labelled with older person's details • completed pathology request form • specimen bag • gloves and apron • clinical waste bag	To maintain older person's dignity, in that you do not have to leave during the procedure. To be organised in advance in order to be efficient. Most catheter bags have a needle-free port which allows the syringe to be connected without the use of a needle. However, some catheter bags do have a port that requires a needle to be used.
Clamp drainage tube with gate clip just below the sampling port on catheter bag. Swab sample port with swab saturated with 70% isopropyl alcohol or spray with 70% isopropyl alcohol. Allow to dry for a minimum of 30 seconds. With syringe (and needle attached if needed) withdraw 20 ml of urine. Remove gate clip.	This is a non-touch technique to maintain as closed a circuit as possible. If there is no urine present in the catheter tubing you may need to wait 15–20 minutes before taking the sample of urine. Do not take a sample out of the catheter bag as it will be contaminated and give a false reading/result.

Place syringe, needle (if used) and urine on clean tray and take to private area such as sluice.	
Transfer 10 ml into sterile container, and pour remainder of urine into clear container. Assess for macroscopic appearance: • cloudy – settlement of sediment and infection • milky – infection, chluria, spermatozoa, urate crystals, insoluble phosphates • blue/green – pseudomonas, bilirubin • pink/red – blood, drugs, beetroot • orange – drugs • yellow and brown – bilirubin • brown/black – blood Assess urine for odour – if left to stand smells of ammonia; if infected smells fishy; if it contains ketones smells sweet. Assess for volume: average output 1500 ml per 24 hours.	To adhere to good recording and documentation legislation and to monitor change.
Test with urinalysis stick by dipping stick into a fresh, well-mixed sample of urine, withdraw stick and wipe along rim of container to remove excess urine, compare with colour chart on side of container for specified time: • presence of glucose – diabetes, Cushing's syndrome, acute pancreatitis • presence of ketones – starvation, diabetes • presence of protein – renal disease, urinary tract infection, congestive heart failure • presence of blood – trauma, infection, renal stones, drugs • presence of bilirubin – hepatic or biliary disease, stale urine • raised urobilinogen – liver disease, haemolytic anaemia	To monitor change. If any abnormalities found, ensure you report to appropriate health care professional so that treatment can begin if appropriate. These are possible indications only.

• presence of nitrites – urinary tract infection • presence of leucocytes – urinary tract infection • pH greater that 7 (acidic) may indicate infection and fever	
Ensure the older person's name, address or ward, and date and time are recorded on pathology request form. Place sealed container in specimen bag with form. If specimen bag is transparent ensure details are not visible through the bag. Send as soon as possible to pathology.	To ensure correct information is given to the laboratory. To preserve patient confidentiality. If kept at room temperature organisms multiply and lead to misinterpretation of results.

6   Care for the older person requiring observation and monitoring

This section focuses on procedures that monitor the physical functioning of the older person, often referred to as measuring and recording the vital signs. This includes the person's body temperature, pulse rate, respiratory rate and blood pressure.

When you measure and record vital signs you are monitoring for signs of abnormalities within the person's homeostatic mechanisms, in order for the appropriate medical or nursing care to be undertaken. Homeostasis is the process by which the human body maintains a constant internal environment, despite external changes. As the person grows older multiple pathology (several different diseases together) is common and therefore homeostasis can be affected. Because the older person is less adaptable and sensation may be reduced, diseases can take longer to show themselves, and the body is slower to mount its defences. Hence, there can be a rapid deterioration. Observation and monitoring of vital signs are therefore extremely important (Caird & Grimley Evans 1995). In order to be able to do this you need to know about the body and how it works. Hence knowledge of anatomy and physiology is crucial. If you are not a registered practitioner, or if you are a lay carer, you should ensure that you are adequately prepared, supervised and aware of the importance of the task (Garrard & Young 1998; NMC 2004a).

BODY TEMPERATURE

Body temperature is the balance between heat from metabolism, muscular activity, and other factors that produce heat, and the heat that is lost through the skin, lungs and body waste. Normal temperature in adults ranges from 36°C to 37.5°C. A stable temperature is important for the proper function of cells, tissues and organs. As we get older, our blood circulation slows and there is a reduction of subcutaneous fat. The body takes longer to adapt to changes in temperature, both internally and externally (Caird & Grimley Evans 1995). The older person may not recognise changes in body temperature, and so respond appropriately by keeping warm, or cooling down, as required. Moreover, the person may become less active as he or she grows older and this will affect body temperature. Low body temperature (hypothermia) may be a problem in cold weather, and may be exacerbated by underlying disease and inadequate and cold housing. A raised body temperature (hyperthermia or pyrexia), may develop in hot weather or as a result of infection.

BLOOD PRESSURE AND PULSE

Blood pressure is the pressure of the blood against the walls of the arteries. It is the result of two forces: the heart creates one as it pumps blood into the arteries and through the circulatory system and the other is the force of the arteries as they resist the blood flow. Blood pressure consists of systolic pressure and diastolic pressure. Systolic pressure is when the left ventricle contracts and is affected by the integrity of the heart and arteries. Diastolic pressure is when the left ventricle relaxes and indicates blood vessel resistance. Blood pressure is measured in millimetres of mercury (mmHg). In younger adults systolic is 90–130 mmHg and diastolic is 60–90 mmHg; in the older person systolic is 140–160 mmHg and diastolic 70–90 mmHg.

The cardiovascular system is also affected by age. Arteries stiffen in the older person, losing their elasticity so that the systolic pressure increases and diastolic pressure falls. There is increased susceptibility to cardiac ischaemia and hence heart attack. The heart of the older person has to pump harder against greater resistance in the arteries and so the heart rate tends to rise. Older adults are more susceptible to heart arrhythmias. The sedentary lifestyle of many older people, together with lifelong dietary habits, may exacerbate the changes that increase the risk of cardiovascular instability (Forman & Wei 1997).

Pulse rate is the wave that occurs when blood is pumped into an already full aorta during ventricular contraction, creating a wave that travels from the heart to the peripheral arteries. The pulse can be palpated at the locations on the body where an artery crosses over bone or firm tissue (see Diagram 7). A person's pulse involves the number of beats per minute (the rate), the pattern or regularity of the beats (rhythm) and also the volume of blood pumped with each beat (strength). Pulse rate in an adult is between 60 and 90 beats per minute, with an average of 80.

RESPIRATORY RATE

Respiration is the exchange of oxygen and carbon dioxide between the atmosphere and the body. Breathing occurs through the work of the diaphragm and chest muscles, and delivers oxygen to the lower respiratory tract and alveoli. Respirations are measured according to rate, rhythm, depth and sound. This reflects the body's metabolic state, diaphragm and chest muscle condition and airway patency. Respiratory rate is a highly sensitive marker when a person's condition is either deteriorating or improving and normal respiratory rate is between 12 and 15 breaths per minute. Each breath includes inspiration and expiration (breathing in and breathing out).

The respiratory system also changes as the person grows older. Ribs lose calcium, while costal cartilage calcifies. The ageing lung becomes less elastic. Arthritic changes in the rib cage tend to make the chest barrel shaped. There is a reduction in lung and breathing capacity. Lower lung volumes mean the older person has to expend more effort during breathing. These changes leave the older person with less reserve capacity to buffer infections such as pneumonia. Natural defences also decline with age. Mucociliary protection of the lower airway is impaired. There is an increased

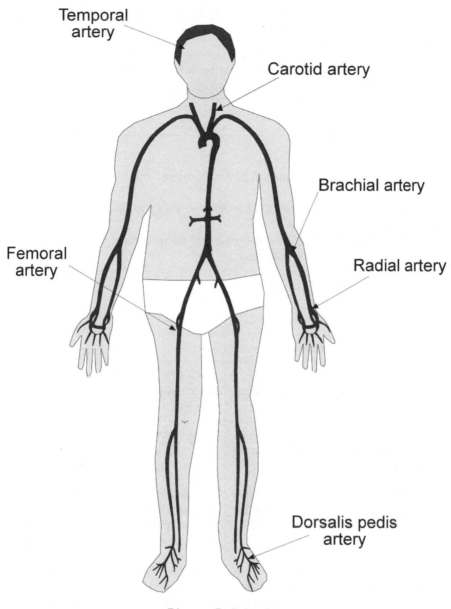

Diagram 7   Pulse sites.

risk of aspiration pneumonia as cough and gag reflexes weaken in the person who has reached older age. Immune function, the body's capacity to fight disease, also declines in the older person, making him or her prone to chest infections, particularly pneumonia and influenza (Polakoff 1997; Coni & Webster 1998).

Procedure Twenty-seven   Measuring and recording temperature

Care requirement
The older person's temperature needs to be monitored and recorded to ensure well-being. Care should be given by an appropriately trained person.

Care objectives
The older person's temperature will be monitored and will remain within acceptable ranges. Appropriate action may be taken if the older person's temperature rises above or falls below acceptable ranges. The older person will understand the reason for the procedure. The older person will feel comfortable.

Care actions	Rationale
See Symbols 1–5, Chapter 1.	
If taking the temperature orally, check whether person has had a hot/cold drink or has smoked in previous 15 minutes.	These affect the temperature of the sub-lingual pocket of tissue activates and may give a false reading.
Open the disposable thermometer without touching the part that will be placed in the person's mouth.	To prevent cross-infection.
Place thermometer under the tongue then ask the older person to close his or her mouth.	This area is in close proximity to the thermoreceptors that respond rapidly to changes in the core temperature. Closed mouth will prevent cool air circulating in mouth.
If taking the temperature under the axilla, place the thermometer lengthwise, dots facing chest wall, arm held against the chest.	This site is considered less desirable as it is not close to major vessels, and skin surface temperatures vary more with changes in the environment.
Leave in place for the correct amount of time, but not too long (1 min oral, 3 min axilla).	To ensure a correct and accurate reading.

Remove thermometer without contaminating hands.	To prevent cross-infection.
Read temperature accurately by counting the number of dots that have changed colour.	
Document and report result.	To plan care.

Procedure Twenty-eight   Measuring and recording temperature using a tympanic thermometer

Care requirement
The older person's temperature needs to be monitored and recorded to ensure well-being. Care should be given by an appropriately trained person.

Care objectives
The older person's temperature will be monitored and will remain within acceptable ranges. Appropriate action may be taken if the older person's temperature rises above or falls below acceptable ranges. The older person will understand the reason for the procedure. The older person will feel comfortable.

Care actions	Rationale
See Symbols 1–5, Chapter 1.	
Cover the thermometer probe with disposable cover without contaminating it.	The probe cover protects the tip of the thermometer and also prevents cross-infection. The cover is also necessary for the functioning of the thermometer.
Gently insert into the ear canal, adjacent to but not touching tympanic membrane according to the manufacturer's instructions.	An infrared light detects heat radiated from the tympanic membrane and provides a digital reading.
Leave thermometer in for correct amount of time – indicated by a bleeping sound.	To ensure correct reading.
Remove thermometer without contaminating hands. Remove probe cover without contaminating hands and discard in clinical waste.	To prevent cross-infection.
Read temperature accurately.	
Document and report result.	To plan care.

Procedure Twenty-nine   Measuring and recording blood pressure

Care requirement
The older person's blood pressure needs to be monitored and recorded to ensure well-being. Care should be given by an appropriately trained person.

Care objectives
The older person's blood pressure will be monitored and will remain within acceptable ranges. Appropriate action may be taken if the older person's blood pressure rises above or falls below acceptable ranges. The older person will understand the reason for the procedure. The older person will feel comfortable.

Care actions	Rationale
See Symbols 1–5, Chapter 1.	
Check for any recent eating, drinking or smoking. Take sphygmomanometer to older person.	Ideally the older person should not eat or drink for half an hour before the measurement is taken, as this might temporarily affect blood pressure. Similarly, the older person should be asked to refrain from smoking for 30 minutes prior to measurement.
Check for recent exercise, to ensure that the older person is adequately rested.	The older person should rest for three minutes if the blood pressure is to be measured when he/she is seated or lying down, and for one minute if a standing measurement is to be taken. This is to minimise the effect of exercise on the blood pressure.
Position the arm of the older person so that it is resting comfortably, with the palm facing up. The arm must be positioned correctly at the level of the heart. A pillow may help to do this.	To ensure an accurate reading is obtained.

Tight clothing that may restrict normal blood flow should be loosened or removed prior to measuring.	Tight clothing may compress the artery and therefore affect the blood pressure reading.
Select the appropriate size of cuff. The length of the bladder within the cuff needs to be at least 80 per cent of the arm circumference.	Incorrect cuff size may give an incorrect reading.
Cuff position, just above elbow, access to ante-cubital fossa (see Diagram 8). The centre of the bladder should be placed over the brachial artery.	Incorrect positioning will give an incorrect reading.
The sphygmomanometer should be placed on a flat surface with the dial/column at your eye level.	To ensure correct reading and so that you have easy viewing of the dial/column.
Perform a radial pulse check to establish the approximate systolic pressure, by inflating the cuff until the radial pulse can no longer be felt. Then deflate the cuff prior to performing the full systolic and diastolic reading.	To give you an estimated systolic pressure. If not deflated the blood pressure will be affected.
Locate the brachial artery (see Diagram 8) and position the stethoscope over it. Ensure the stethoscope is functioning and positioned correctly in the ears.	Do not tuck the diaphragm under the cuff as this may occlude the brachial artery when the cuff is inflated.
The cuff should be inflated to 20–30 mmHg above the previously estimated systolic reading.	To help you obtain an accurate reading.
Deflate the cuff at 33 mmHg per second and in a controlled manner.	At a too slow rate venous congestion and arm pain can develop, resulting in a false low reading. A too fast deflation will result in a false high reading.

Take note of the systolic and diastolic pressures correctly. Systolic pressure is the first Kortkoff (thudding) sound you will hear, and the diastolic is where the sound disappears (fifth Kortkoff). Once sounds have disappeared, open the valve fully, to completely deflate the cuff and remove from the patient's arm. Any restrictive clothing is replaced and the patient is helped to a comfortable resting position after the procedure.	To ensure an accurate reading.
Clean stethoscope ear pieces as necessary.	If a stethoscope is used by or for more than one person, ear pieces and bell should be cleaned between uses to prevent cross-infection by wiping with an alcohol wipe and allowing to dry for a minimum of 30 seconds.

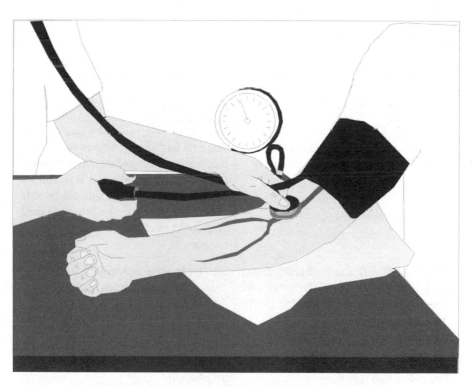

Diagram 8 Blood pressure cuff and brachial artery position.

Procedure Thirty   Measuring and recording pulse

Care requirement
The older person's pulse needs to be monitored and recorded to ensure well-being. Care should be given by an appropriately trained person.

Care objectives
The older person's pulse will be monitored and will remain within acceptable ranges. Appropriate action may be taken if the older person's pulse rises above or falls below acceptable ranges. The older person will understand the reason for the procedure. The older person will feel comfortable.

Care actions	Rationale
See Symbols 1–5, Chapter 1.	
Check for recent exercise and that the person's arm is resting comfortably.	Recent exercise, and discomfort, will cause an increase in the pulse rate.
Locate radial pulse accurately (see Diagram 8).	This is the usual site of choice as it is easily felt here.
Using the first and second fingers, lightly but firmly compress the artery	The first and second fingers are used as they are sensitive and do not have pulses of their own like the thumb. If you do not compress enough you will not be able to feel the pulse; if you press too hard you could occlude the artery or harm the person.
Using watch with a second hand, count the beats for 30 seconds (if regular) and note rate, volume, rhythm and strength. You will need to double the figure to obtain the pulse rate per minute. If irregular count for one minute.	Sufficient time is required in order to detect any irregularities or defects.
Document and report.	To plan care.

Procedure Thirty-one   Measuring and recording respiratory rate

Care requirement
The older person's respiration needs to be monitored and recorded to ensure well-being. Care should be given by an appropriately trained person.

Care objectives
The older person's respiration will be monitored and will remain within acceptable ranges. Appropriate action may be taken if the older person's respirations rise above or fall below acceptable ranges. The older person will understand the reason for the procedure. The older person will feel comfortable.

Care actions	Rationale
See Symbols 1–5, Chapter 1.	
Check for any recent exercise and ensure the person is comfortable.	Recent exercise, and discomfort, will cause an increase in the respiratory rate.
Observe the rise and fall of the chest; each rise and fall counts as one respiration. It is best to try and ensure that the person is unaware you are observing their breathing.	If the person is aware that you are counting their respiratory rate they subconsciously change the pattern of their breathing. A good tip is to count it directly after the pulse rate. You can explain this to the older person when you gain consent at the beginning of the procedure.
If respirations are regular, even and unlaboured, count for 30 seconds and then double to obtain number of respirations per minute. If abnormal in any way, you should count for one minute. Observe the sound, depth and pattern of respirations.	Sufficient time is required in order to detect any irregularities or defects.
Document and report.	To plan care.

7   Care for the older person at the end of his or her life

The biological process of ageing means an increased inability to resist death (Coni & Webster 1998). Eighty per cent of deaths occur in people aged 65 and over. Sixty-five per cent of deaths occur in women over the age of 75. Fifty-four per cent of deaths take place in National Health Service hospitals, 13 per cent in care homes and 4 per cent in hospices. Twenty per cent of deaths occur in older people's own homes. Ischaemic heart disease, cancer, stroke and respiratory diseases are the leading causes of death in older people in England. Many deaths follow periods of disability and dependency. The older person who has dementia may endure a protracted period, lasting some weeks, of being near death, and in distress, with or without pain (Baines 1995). For the older person's family, death may bring shock because of its suddenness, or it may follow a long period of caring with consequent emotional and physical stress.

QUALITY OF LIFE FOR THE DYING OLDER PERSON

Care for the older person who is dying focuses on the older person, his or her family and significant others. The aim is to assist the older person and family to have quality in the remaining life they have together. Care should be directed towards helping the older person to achieve and experience whatever is important to him or her, as far as possible and practicable. The process of dying may be sudden, or it may take weeks or even months. In the latter case your role may be to help the older person to remain as mobile as possible. This could involve help to get out and about by the use of a wheelchair and possibly a car. As the older person's condition progresses, ensuring the older person is as comfortable as possible will also comfort the family. They too need support as they come to terms with their coming loss.

Caring for the dying older person may involve the carer carrying out very many of the procedures listed in this book. Additionally, the carer may also need more specialist help in controlling the older person's symptoms as far as is possible. These may include pain, anxiety and depression, restlessness and confusion, nausea and vomiting, anorexia, constipation, breathlessness, any offensive fungating tumours and bowel obstruction, and will involve specialist care. You will need to seek help and advice from the appropriate professional. Many older people will prefer to die at home. This may be possible with the extra support of community nurses, Marie Curie Cancer Care Nurses and Macmillan Nurses. Marie Curie Cancer Care Nurses can provide care at home by day or night, giving the carer a break, while Macmillan Nurses offer symptom control and emotional support.

CARING FOR THE WHOLE PERSON

Care should constantly be re-assessed and evaluated and the older person's comfort monitored. Changes may occur rapidly, and will need to be addressed. The older person's needs and desires should be paramount. While specialist help is important, the older person who is dying may appreciate the seemingly small comforts that show you care and that you are there alongside him or her as life reaches an end. The smallest attentions, such as a sip of water to moisten the lips, the moving of a pillow, shading the light, holding the hand, are crucial as the older person's life draws to an end. If possible, and if the older person wants it, someone should stay by the bedside. As the carer you should be guided by knowledge and understanding of the older person and family, built up over the time you are together, and listen for clues about how care should proceed.

The spiritual dimension of care for the older person comes to the fore in caring for the older person who is dying. Although illness and ageing generally raise questions of meaning about the nature and purpose of life, these questions are highlighted as the end of life approaches as a reality. The older person's and family's religious faith or personal meanings are particularly relevant. You as the carer should have some understanding of the varieties of religious belief and what they mean to the older person who may hold these beliefs. In the UK in 1998, despite the decline in church membership, only one in ten people said they did not believe in God, and one in five people said that they had no doubt that God exists (Office for National Statistics 2000: 219). In 1990 more than six and a half million people were members of a Christian church, half a million people belonged to Islam, a quarter of a million were adherents of Sikhism, 140 000 belonged to the Hindu religion, and 101 000 were Jewish. You may need to find out how both the older person and family can be supported, possibly by the assistance of a chaplain or faith minister. Sensitivity in recognising the complexity of the spiritual dimension in the life of the individual is vital.

AFTER DEATH

After death at home or hospital a doctor should see the body to confirm and certify death. If death is unexpected you may need to inform the family. You will need sensitivity to do this. The family may like to spend time with the body, and the room should stay unchanged while this happens. Privacy might be needed for the family at this time and thus the carer will need discretion. It is important for the carer to show sensitivity and understanding towards the bereaved. This is where your relationship with the family will be particularly important. Small, seemingly insignificant, attentions show you care and have understanding and compassion. For example, have tissues available, perhaps offer a cup of tea or other drink, ensure there are comfortable chairs, that debris is removed and that the room is peaceful.

Religious considerations should be observed in laying out the body. You should treat the body of the deceased older person with respect. If you are working with a colleague to lay out the body you should maintain silence. If you do need to talk to your partner, then do so minimally and quietly.

Formalities will need to be carried out in registering the death and preparing for the funeral. It will help the family if you can support them in doing this by informing them whom to contact. It may also be helpful if you can advise them on what bereavement support may be available. Above all, be sensitive to the family's individual needs.

Procedure Thirty-two   Caring for the body of the older person following death

Care requirements
The older person has died. Care should be given by an appropriately trained person.

Care objectives
To confirm death and to prepare the body for removal, according to the choice of the deceased older person. To support the family/friends of the deceased older person.

Care actions	Rationale
See Symbols 1–5, Chapter 1.	The deceased person should be treated with respect.
Inform doctor/senior nurse.	Confirmation of death should be confirmed by a doctor or a senior nurse who has been trained in certification. A doctor who has attended the deceased person during the last illness is required to give a medical certificate of the cause of death. The certificate requires the doctor to state the last date on which he/she saw the deceased alive and whether he/she has seen the body after death. Confirmation of death should be recorded in the older person's notes.
Inform next of kin/family and friends. Discuss cultural/religious preferences with regard to preparation of body. Be sensitive to family/friends if they desire to sit with deceased person. Ensure privacy and explain all procedures. Check previous documentation.	To ensure the family/friends are informed and give valid consent. To support their bereavement and provide sensitive care. To gain trust and confidence of family and friends. To assist participation. To support the making of funeral arrangements. To offer support of hospital chaplain or local minister and/or take formal account of any specific religious/cultural practices. To take into account previously made plans.

As soon as possible lay older person on his/her back. Remove all but one pillow. To prevent the mouth from falling open, support the jaw by placing a pillow or rolled up towel on chest under jaw. Remove any devices or aids attached to the older person as long as post-mortem is not required. Straighten limbs and close eyes by applying light pressure for 30 seconds.	To maintain the deceased older person's dignity. Rigor mortis occurs 2-4 hours after death.
Inform staff and other patients.	To ensure continuity of care and support for family/friends, and for other patients.
If agreed by family/friends, and if culturally appropriate, begin to prepare the body of the deceased older person.	To take formal account of any specific religious/cultural practices. (Some religious traditions have specific practices with regard to who may touch the body after death.) To maintain dignity of deceased person. To provide support, both physical and emotional.
Collect equipment on trolley: • bowl, soap, towel, two face cloths • razor – electric or disposable – comb, nail scissors • equipment for care of mouth, including toothbrush, sponge swabs/foam sticks • equipment for cleaning dentures • identification labels • Documents required for law or hospital policies (e.g. notification-of-death cards) • gloves and apron • clean clothes or shroud to dress older person, as required by family/friends • body bag if required • cottonwool balls if required • wound pack if required • tape • valuables or property book • clinical waste bag • linen skip • hoist or slings if required to move body	To respect the dignity of the deceased body, in that you will not have to leave during the procedure. A body bag is used according to local policy, if bodily fluids are leaking or if deceased person is infectious.

Drain the bladder by pressing the lower abdomen.	Because fluids may still be excreted from the body after death.
Pack leaking orifices with cottonwool, remove any drains, tubes and catheters if no post-mortem required. Cover wounds with wound dressing and secure with occlusive dressing. Cover drain sites with occlusive dressing.	Open wounds and leaking orifices pose a hazard to anyone coming into contact with the body. If a post-mortem is required, leave all tubes and drains *in situ*.
Taking account of religious and cultural practices, wash the older person as in Procedure Two (p. 34) if required. Shave the older person if necessary. Clean the mouth with sponge swabs ensuring it is free from debris and secretions. Clean dentures and place in mouth if possible.	For reasons of hygiene and dignity. Family/friends may like to be involved as part of grieving process. Some religious traditions have specific practices with regard to who may touch the body after death.
Taking account of the wishes of family/friends, remove all jewellery in the presence of a witness. Document any jewellery remaining on the deceased person (e.g. wedding ring) on the notification of death form. Record jewellery and other valuables in property book and store according to local policy.	To meet legal requirements and wishes of family/friends.
Dress older person in chosen clothing. If required as part of policy, label one wrist and one ankle with identification labels. Complete any documents requiring notification of death and tape securely to shroud or clothing.	To ensure correct identification in mortuary/funeral directors' premises.

Remove bottom sheet from bed and introduce mortuary sheet by rolling older person from side to side as described in Procedure One (p. 31). Fold top of mortuary sheet over deceased person's face. Fold mortuary sheet over right side, and bottom of mortuary sheet over older person's feet and lower limbs. Fold mortuary sheet over left side and ensure that all parts of the body are well covered. Secure the sheet with tape. Place the body in a body bag if required. Tape identification card to mortuary sheet. Cover with sheet.	To prevent damage to the body and distress or health hazard to others. To ensure correct identification in mortuary. To maintain dignity.
Ask porters/funeral directors to remove body. Screen off appropriate area.	The body decomposes rapidly in hot weather and heated rooms. Prevent bacterial hazard by cooling body in mortuary. Screening the area may prevent further distress to others.
If in hospital/care home pack up property. Transfer property to family/friends or appropriate department.	As a legal record. Formalities require appropriate documentation.
	Ask family/friends if they have any requirements, in order to support them. Document time of death in appropriate documentation, recording names of those present and names of people informed. Transfer documentation to relevant administration. This is a legal record. Formalities require appropriate documentation.

References and further reading

Age Concern (2006) *Hungry to be Heard*, Age Concern, London.

Baillie, L. (2005) *Developing Practical Nursing Skills*, Arnold, London.

Baines, M.J. (1995) Terminal illness, in D.J. Weatherall, J.G.G. Ledingham & D.A. Warrell, (eds), *Oxford Textbook of Medicine*, vol. 3, Oxford University Press, Oxford, pp. 4349–60.

Baker, F., Smith, L. & Stead, L. (1999a) Practical procedures for nurses: giving a blanket bath – 1, 21.1, *Nursing Times*, **95** (3).

Baker, F., Smith, L. & Stead, L. (1999b) Practical procedures for nurses: giving a blanket bath – 2, 21.2, *Nursing Times*, **95** (4).

Baker, F., Smith, L. & Stead, L. (1999c) Practical procedures for nurses: washing a patient's hair in bed – 22.1, *Nursing Times*, **95** (5).

Beauchamp, T. & Childress, J. (2001) *Principles of Biomedical Ethics*, 4th edn, Oxford University Press, Oxford.

Beevers, G., Lip, G. & O'Brien, E. (2001a) Blood pressure measurement. Part 1: Sphygmomanometry: factors common to all techniques. *British Medical Journal*, **322**, 981–5.

Beevers, G., Lip, G. & O'Brien, E. (2001b) Blood pressure measurement. Part 2: Conventional sphygmomanometry: a technique of auscultatory blood pressure measurement. *British Medical Journal*, **322**, 1043–7.

Best, C. (2005) Caring for the patient with a nasogastric tube. *Nursing Standard*, **20** (3), 59–65.

Betts, M. & Mowbray, C. (2005) The falling and fallen person and emergency handling, in J. Smith (ed.), *The Guide to the Handling of People*, 5th edn, Backcare/RCN/National Back Exchange, Middlesex.

Birch, S. & Coggins, T. (2003) No-rinse one step bed bath: effects on the occurrences of skin tears in a long term care setting. *Ostomy Wound Management*, **19** (1), 64–7.

Bond, J., Coleman, P. & Pearce, S. (eds) (1999) *Ageing in Society*, 2nd edn, Sage, London.

Bond, S. (ed.) (1997) *Eating Matters*, Newcastle upon Tyne, Centre for Health Services Research, University of Newcastle.

Bowling, T. (2004) *Nutritional Support for Adults and Children: a handbook for hospital practice*, Radcliffe Medical Press, Oxford.

Caird, F.I. & Grimley Evans, J. (1995) Medicine in old age, in D.J. Weatherall, J.G.G. Ledingham & D.A. Warrell (eds), *Oxford Textbook of Medicine*, vol. 3, Oxford University Press, Oxford, pp. 4333–6.

Centaur (1999) *Load Management Theory and Client Handling Techniques*. Centaur Training Ltd, Cleveland, Ohio.

Clinical Resource Efficiency Support Team (CREST) (2004) Guidelines for the management of enteral tube feeding in adults, www.crestni.org.uk (accessed 3 November 2005).

Colley, W. (1999a) Practical procedures for nurses: constipation – 1, causes and assessment, 27.1, *Nursing Times*, **95** (20).

Colley, W. (1999b) Practical procedures for nurses: constipation – 2, treatment, 27.2, *Nursing Times*, **95** (21).

Commission for Healthcare Audit and Inspection (2006) *Living Well in Later Life*, Commission for Healthcare Audit and Inspection, London.

Coni, N. & Webster, S. (1998) *Lecture Notes on Geriatrics*, Blackwell Science, Oxford.

Department of Health (DoH) (1999) *Drug Tariff*, HMSO, London.

Department of Health (DoH) (2001a) *National Service Framework for Older People*, DoH, London.

Department of Health, Standing Nursing and Midwifery Advisory Committee (2001b) *Caring for Older People: a Nursing Priority*, DoH, London.

Department of Health (DoH) (2001c) *The Essence of Care*, DoH, London.

Department of Health (DoH) (2001d) Standard principles for preventing hospital-acquired infections. *Journal of Hospital Infection*, **47**, 21–37.

Department of Health (DoH) (2001e) *Reference Guide to Seeking Consent: working with older people*, DOH, London.

Department of Health (DoH) (2001f) *Reference Guide to Consent for Examination or Treatment*, DOH, London.

Department of Health (DoH) (2003) *Infection Control, Prevention of Healthcare-associated Infection in Primary and Community Care*, National Institute for Clinical Excellence, London.

Department of Health (DoH) (2005a) *A Simple Guide to* Clostridium difficile, DoH, London, www.dh.gov.uk/hcai.

Department of Health (DoH) (2005b) Infection caused by *Clostridium difficile*. Letter from the Chief Medical Officer and Chief Nursing Officer. Ref: PL CMO (2005) 6; PL CNO (2005) 5.

Department of Health (DoH) (2005c) *Saving lives*, DoH, London.

Department of Health (DoH) (2006) *A New Ambition for Old Age*, DoH, London.

Dimond, B (2005) *Legal Aspects of Nursing*, Pearson Education, Harlow.

Dougherty, L. & Lister, S. (eds) (2004) *Manual of Clinical Nursing Procedures*, 6th edn, Blackwell Science, Oxford.

Eliopoulos, C. (2001) *Gerontological Nursing*, 5th edn, Lippincott, Philadelphia.

Field, D. (1998a) Practical procedures for nurses: mouth care – 1, 19.1, *Nursing Times*, **94** (7).

Field, D. (1998b) Practical procedures for nurses: mouth care – 2, 19.2, *Nursing Times*, **94** (8).

Forman, D. & Wei, J. (1997) Congestive heart failure in the elderly, in J. Wei & M. Sheehan (eds), *Geriatric Medicine,* Oxford University Press, Oxford, pp. 67–79.

Fullbrook, P. (1993) Core temperature measurement in adults: a literature review, *Journal of Advanced Nursing*, **18** (9), 1451–60.

Garrard, G. & Young, C. (1998) Suboptimal care of patients before admission to intensive care. *British Medical Journal*, **316**, 1841–2.

Gill, D. (1999a) Practical procedures for nurses: stool specimen – 1, Assessment, 31.1, *Nursing Times*, **95** (25).

Gill, D. (1999b) Practical procedures for nurses: stool specimen – 2, Collection, 31.2, *Nursing Times*, **95** (26).

Gillespie, A. & Curzio, J. (1998) Blood pressure measurement: assessing staff knowledge. *Nursing Standard*, **12** (23), 35–7.

Gould, D. (2002) Hand decontamination. *Nursing Times*, **98** (46), 48–9.

Grimley Evans, J., Franklin Williams, T., Lynn Beattie, B., Michel, J.-P. & Wilcock, G.K. (2000) *Oxford Textbook of Geriatric Medicine*, Oxford University Press, Oxford.

Hampton, S. (2004) Caring for the skin of older residents: a practical guide. *Nursing and Residential Care*, **6** (7), 326–9.

Handbook of Nursing Procedures (2001) Springhouse, Pennsylvania.

Harrison, S. (2005) Deaths prompt alert over nasogastric tube insertion. *Nursing Standard*, **19** (25), 7.

Hayes, A. & Yohannes, A. (1998) Keeping active, in J. Marr & B. Kershaw (eds), *Caring for Older People*, Arnold, London, pp. 71–88.

Health and Safety Commission (HSC) (1998) *Manual Handling in the Health Services*, HSE Books, Suffolk.

Health and Safety Executive, Health Services Advisory Committee (1992) *Safe Disposal of Clinical Waste*, HMSO, Sheffield.

Health and Safety Executive (2005) *Back Pain and Injury at Work*, HSE Books, London.

Help the Aged (2005) *Preventing Falls: don't mention the f-word!* Help the Aged, London.

Henderson, V. & Nite, G. (1978) *Principles and Practice of Nursing*, Macmillan, London.

Hill, M. & Grim, C. (1991) How to take a precise blood pressure. *American Journal of Nursing*, **91** (2), 38–42.

Holmes, D. (1999) *The Guide to the Handling of Patients*, rev. 4th edn, NBPA/RCN, Middlesex.

Jevon, P. & Jevon, M. (2001a) Practical procedures for nurses: using a tympanic thermometer, 56.1, *Nursing Times*, **97** (9), 43–4.

Jevon, P. & Jevon, M. (2001b) Practical procedures for nurses: facial shaving, 57.1, *Nursing Times*, **97** (11).

Johnson, C. (2005) Manual handling risk assessment theory and practice, in J. Smith (ed), *The Guide to the Handling of People*, 5th edn. Backcare/RCN/National Back Exchange, Middlesex.

Johnson, F. (1997) Disposable gloves: research findings on use in practice. *Nursing Standard*, **11** (16), 39–40.

Kenwood, G., Hodgetts, T. & Castle, N. (2001) Time to put the R back into TPR. *Nursing Times*, **97** (40).

Leggatt, P. (1999) *The Guide to the Handling of Patients*, rev. 4th edn, NBPA/RCN, Middlesex, Ch 5

Lennard-Jones, J.E. (1992) *A Positive Approach to Nutrition as Treatment*, King's Fund, London.

Lewis-Byers, K. & Thayner, D. (2002) An evaluation of two incontinence care protocols in a long-term care setting. *Ostomy Wound Management*, **48** (12), 44–51.

Macaulay, M. (1997) Urinary drainage systems, in S. Fillingham & J. Douglas (eds), *Urological Nursing*, 2nd edn, Bailliere Tindall, London, pp. 90–130.

McWhirter, J.P. & Pennington, C.R. (1994) Incidence and recognition of malnutrition in hospital. *British Medical Journal*, **308**, 945–8.

Mallett, J. & Dougherty, L. (eds) (2000) *Manual of Clinical Nursing Procedures*, Blackwell Science, Oxford.

Malnutrition Advisory Group (2003) Press release. www.bapen.org.uk/mag.htm (accessed 24 October 2005).

Mandelstam, M. (2002) *Manual Handling in Health and Social Care*, Jessica Kingsley, London.

Mathey, M.-F. A. M., Siebelink, E., de Graaf, C. & Van Staveren, W.A. (2001) Flavor enhancement of food improves dietary intake and nutritional status of elderly nursing home residents. *Journals of Gerontology Series A: Biological Sciences and Medical Sciences*, **56**, M200–5.

Moore, L.W. & Miller, M. (2003) Older men's experience of living with severe visual impairment. *Journal of Advanced Nursing*, **43** (1), 10–18.

Moppett, S. & Parker, M. (1999) Practical procedures for nurses: insertion of a suppository, 29.1, *Nursing Times*, **95** (23).

National Institute for Clinical Excellence (2004) *Falls: The Assessment and Prevention of Falls in Older People*, National Institute for Clinical Excellence, London.

National Patient Safety Agency (2005) Reducing the harm caused by misplaced nasogastric feeding tubes, www.npsa.hns.uk (accessed 24 October 2005).

Nearney, L. (1998a) Practical procedures for nurses: last offices – 1, 14.1, *Nursing Times*, **94** (26).

Nearney, L. (1998b) Practical procedures for nurses: last offices – 2, 14.2, *Nursing Times*, **94** (27).

Nearney, L. (1998c) Practical procedures for nurses: last offices – 3, 14.3, *Nursing Times*, **94** (28).

NHS Plus (2006a) www.nhsplus.nhs.uk/your_health/backpain.asp (accessed 27 March 2006).

NHS Plus (2006b) www.nhsplus.nhs.uk/nhsstaff/manual.asp (accessed 27 March 2006).

Nicol, M., Bavin, C., Bedford-Turner, S., Cronin, P. & Rawlings-Anderson, K. (2005) *Essential Nursing Skills*, 2nd edn, Elsevier Mosby, London.

Nightingale, F. (1860) *Notes on Nursing*, Harrison, London.

Norgine Pharmaceuticals Limited (2000) *The Bristol Stool Form Scale*, Norgine Pharmaceuticals Limited, Harefield.

Nursing and Midwifery Council (NMC) (2004a) *The NMC Code of Professional Conduct: Standards for Conduct, Performance and Ethics*, NMC, London.

Nursing and Midwifery Council (NMC) (2004b) *Guidelines for Records and Record Keeping*, NMC, London.

Ochs, G. & Castaldi, P. (2001) *Fundamentals of Nursing*, Mosby, St Louis, Missouri.

Office for National Statistics (2000) *Social Trends*, 30th edn.

O'Donnell, L. J. D., Virjee, J. & Heaton, K. W. (1990) Detection of pseudodiarrhoea by simple clinical assessment of intestinal transit rate. *British Medical Journal* **300**, 439–40.

O'Toole, S. (1997) Disposable gloves. *Professional Nurse*, **13**, 184–90.

Papoola, M., Jenkins, L. & Griffin, O. (2005) Caring for the foot mobile: holistic foot and nail management. *Holistic Nursing Practice*, **19** (5), 222–7.

Penzer, R. & Finch, M. (2001) Promoting healthy skin in older people. *Nursing Older People*, **13** (8), 22–8.

Perry, A. & Potter, P. (2004) *Clinical Nursing Skills and Techniques*, 6th edn, Elsevier Mosby, Philadelphia.

Phillips, G. (1999) Microbiological aspects of clincial waste. *Journal of Hospital Infection*, **41**, 1–6.

Polakoff, D. (1997) Pneumonia in the elderly, in J. Wei & M. Sheehan (eds), *Geriatric Medicine*, Oxford University Press, Oxford, pp. 160–9.

Pomfret, I. (2000) Catheter care in the community. *Nursing Standard*, **14** (27), 46–51.

Rollins, H. (1997) A nose for trouble. *Nursing Times*, **93** (8), 66–7.

Roper, N., Logan, W. & Tierney, A. (1985) *The Elements of Nursing*, 2nd edn, Churchill Livingstone, Edinburgh.

Ross, S. (1999) Rationalising the purchase and use of gloves in health care. *British Journal of Nursing*, **8** (5), 279–87.

Royal College of Nursing (RCN) (1996) *Hazards of Nursing: Personal Injuries at Work*, RCN, London.

Royal College of Nursing (RCN) (2001) *Pressure Ulcer Risk Assessment and Prevention*, RCN, London.

Royal College of Nursing (RCN) (2003) *Manual Handling Assessments in Hospitals and the Community*, RCN, London.

Royal College of Nursing (RCN) (2004) *Good Practice in Infection Control, Guidance for Nursing Staff*, RCN, London.

Royal College of Nursing Institute (1998) *Clinical Practice Guidelines: the management of patients with venous leg ulcers*, RCN Institute, Centre for Evidence Based Nursing, University of York and the School of Nursing, Midwifery and Health Visiting, University of Manchester.

Royal College of Physicians (2002) *Nutrition and Patients: a doctor's responsibility*, RCP, London.

Ruszala, S. (2005) Controversial techniques, in J. Smith (ed), *The Guide to the Handling of People*, 5th edn. Backcare/RCN/National Back Exchange, Middlesex.

Ryan, T. (1995) Diseases of the skin, in D.J. Weatherall, J.G.G. Ledingham & D.A. Warrell (eds), *Oxford Textbook of Medicine*, vol. 3, Oxford University Press, Oxford, pp. 3705–811.

Semple, M. & Elley, K. (1998a) Practical procedures for nurses: catheter specimen of urine, 16.1, *Nursing Times*, **94** (30).

Semple, M. & Elley, K. (1999a) Practical procedures for nurses: collecting a mid-stream specimen of urine, 20.1, *Nursing Times*, **95** (2).

Sheehan, M. (1997) Approach to the older person, In J. Wei & M. Sheehan (eds), *Geriatric Medicine*, Oxford University Press, Oxford, pp. 1–12.

Smith, J. (ed.) (2005) *The Guide to the Handling of People*, 5th edn, Backcare/RCN/NBE, Middlesex.

Smith-Temple J. & Young Johnson, J. (2002) *Nurses' Guide to Clinical Procedures*, Lippincott, Philadelphia.

Storr, J. & Clayton Kent, S. (2004) Hand hygiene. *Nursing Standard*, **80** (40), 45–51.

Strawbridge, W. J., Wallhagen, M. I., Shema, S. J. & Kaplan, G. A. (2000) Negative consequences of hearing impairment in old age: a longitudinal analysis. *The Gerontologist*, **40** (3), 320–6.

Thibodeau, G. A. & Patton, K. T. (eds) (2004) *Structure and Function of the Body*, 12th edn, Mosby, St Louis, Missouri.

Thomas, S. (2005) Sitting to standing, in J. Smith (ed.), *The Guide to the Handling of People*, 5th edn, Backcare/RCN/NBE, Middlesex.

Torrance, C. & Elley, K. (1997a) Practical procedures for nurses: assessing pulse – 1, 3.1, *Nursing Times*, **93** (41).

Torrance, C. & Elley, K. (1997b) Practical procedures for nurses: assessing pulse – 2, 3.2, *Nursing Times*, **93** (42).

Torrance, C. & Elley, K. (1997c) Practical procedures for nurses: breathing, technique and observation – 1, 4.1, *Nursing Times*, **93** (43).

Torrance, C. & Elley, K. (1997d) Practical procedures for nurses: breathing, technique and observation – 2, 4.2, *Nursing Times*, **93** (44).

Torrance, C. & Semple, M. (1997a) Practical procedures for nurses: blood pressure management; equipment, 2.1, *Nursing Times*, **93** (38).

Torrance, C. & Semple, M. (1997b) Practical procedures for nurses: blood pressure management; the patient, 2.2, *Nursing Times*, **93** (39).

Torrance, C. & Semple, M. (1997c) Practical procedures for nurses: blood pressure management; procedure, 2.3, *Nursing Times*, **93** (40).

Torrance, C. & Semple, M. (1998a) Practical procedures for nurses: recording temperature – 1, 6.1, *Nursing Times*, **94** (2).

Torrance, C. & Semple, M. (1998b) Practical procedures for nurses: recording temperature – 2, 6.2, *Nursing Times*, **94** (3).

Wanless, D. (2002) Securing our future: taking a long-term view: final report. http:www.hm-treasury.gov.uk/consultation/wanless (accessed 24 October 2005).

Watts, A. (1998) Practical procedures for nurses 17.2: Eye care – 2, Cleansing the eyelids. *Nursing Times*, **94** (38).

Wilde, M. (1997) Long-term indwelling catheter care: conceptualizing the research/urinary base. *Journal of Advanced Nursing*, **25** (6), 1252–61.

Wilson, J. (1997) Control and prevention of infection in catheter care. *Nurse prescriber/Community Nurse*, **3** (5), 39–40.

Woollons, S. (1996) Temperature measurement devices. *Professional Nurse*, **11** (8), 541–7.

Workman, B. & Bennett, C. (2002) *Key Nursing Skills*, Whurr, London.

Index